Third Edition

Health Promotion and Public Health for Nursing Students

Daryl Evans
Dina Coutsaftiki
C. Patricia Fathers

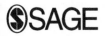

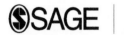

Learning Matters
An imprint of SAGE Publications Ltd
1 Oliver's Yard
55 City Road
London EC1Y 1SP

SAGE Publications Inc.
2455 Teller Road
Thousand Oaks, California 91320

SAGE Publications India Pvt Ltd
B 1/I 1 Mohan Cooperative Industrial Area
Mathura Road
New Delhi 110 044

SAGE Asia-Pacific Pte Ltd
3 Church Street
#10–04 Samsung Hub
Singapore 049483

© Daryl Evans, Dina Coutsaftiki and C. Patricia Fathers

First published in 2011
Second edition published in 2014
Third edition published in 2017

Editor: Alex Clabburn
Development editor: Eleanor Rivers
Production controller: Chris Marke
Project management: Deer Park Productions
Marketing manager: Tamara Navaratnam
Cover design: Wendy Scott
Typeset by: C&M Digitals (P) Ltd, Chennai, India
Printed and bound by
CPI Group (UK) Ltd, Croydon, CR0 4YY

Library of Congress Control Number: 2016960202

British Library Cataloguing in Publication data

A catalogue record for this book is available from the British Library

ISBN 978-1-4739-7785-3 (pbk)
ISBN 978-1-4739-7784-6 (hbk)

At SAGE we take sustainability seriously. Most of our products are printed in the UK using FSC papers and boards. When we print overseas we ensure sustainable papers are used as measured by the PREPS grading system. We undertake an annual audit to monitor our sustainability.

Health Promotion and Public Health for Nursing Students

Sara Miller McCune founded SAGE Publishing in 1965 to support the dissemination of usable knowledge and educate a global community. SAGE publishes more than 1000 journals and over 800 new books each year, spanning a wide range of subject areas. Our growing selection of library products includes archives, data, case studies and video. SAGE remains majority owned by our founder and after her lifetime will become owned by a charitable trust that secures the company's continued independence.

Los Angeles | London | New Delhi | Singapore | Washington DC | Melbourne

Contents

Transforming Nursing Practice is a series tailor-made for pre-registration student nurses. Each book in the series is:

- ○ Affordable
- ○ Mapped to the NMC Standards and Essential Skills Clusters
- ○ Full of active learning features
- ○ Focused on applying theory to practice

Each book addresses a core topic and has been carefully developed to be simple to use, quick to read and written in clear language.

> An invaluable series of books that explicitly relates to the NMC standards.
> Each book covers a different topic that students need to explore in order
> to develop into a qualified nurse... I would recommend this series to all
> pre-registration nursing students whatever their field or year of study
>
> **Linda Robson**
> **Senior Lecturer, Edge Hill University**
>
> The set of books is an excellent resource for students. The series is small,
> easily portable and valuable. I use the whole set on a regular basis.
>
> **Fiona Davies**
> **Senior Nurse Lecturer/Stage 1 Leader/Admissions Tutor, University of Derby**
>
> I recommend the SAGE/Learning Matters series to all my students
> as they are relevant and concise. Please keep up the good work.
>
> **Thomas Beary**
> **Senior Lecturer in Mental Health Nursing, University of Hertfordshire**

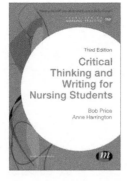

Third Edition
Critical Thinking and Writing for Nursing Students
Bob Price
Anne Harrington

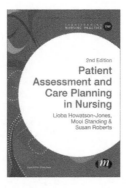

2nd Edition
Patient Assessment and Care Planning in Nursing
Lioba Howatson-Jones,
Mooi Standing &
Susan Roberts

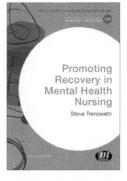

Promoting Recovery in Mental Health Nursing
Steve Trenoweth

CORE KNOWLEDGE TITLES:

Becoming a Registered Nurse: Making the Transition to Practice

Communication and Interpersonal Skills in Nursing (3rd Ed)

Contexts of Contemporary Nursing (2nd Ed)

Getting into Nursing (2nd Ed)

Health Promotion and Public Health for Nursing Students (3rd Ed)

Introduction to Medicines Management in Nursing

Law and Professional Issues in Nursing (3rd Ed)

Leadership, Management and Team Working in Nursing (2nd Ed)

Learning Skills for Nursing Students

Medicines Management in Children's Nursing

Microbiology and Infection Prevention and Control for Nursing Students

Nursing and Collaborative Practice (2nd Ed)

Nursing and Mental Health Care

Nursing in Partnership with Patients and Carers

Palliative and End of Life Care in Nursing

Passing Calculations Tests for Nursing Students (3rd Ed)

Pathophysiology and Pharmacology for Nursing Students

Patient Assessment and Care Planning in Nursing (2nd Ed)

Patient Safety and Managing Risk in Nursing

Psychology and Sociology in Nursing (2nd Ed)

Successful Practice Learning for Nursing Students (2nd Ed)

Understanding Ethics in Nursing Students

Using Health Policy in Nursing Practice

What is Nursing? Exploring Theory and Practice (3rd Ed)

PERSONAL AND PROFESSIONAL LEARNING SKILLS TITLES:

Clinical Judgement and Decision Making for Nursing Students (2nd Ed)

Critical Thinking and Writing for Nursing Students (3rd Ed)

Evidence-based Practice in Nursing (3rd Ed)

Information Skills for Nursing Students

Reflective Practice in Nursing (3rd Ed)

Succeeding in Essays, Exams and OSCEs for Nursing Students

Succeeding in Literature Reviews and Research Project Plans for Nursing Students (2nd Ed)

Successful Professional Portfolios for Nursing Students (2nd Ed)

Understanding Research for Nursing Students (3rd Ed)

MENTAL HEALTH NURSING TITLES:

Assessment and Decision Making in Mental Health Nursing

Engagement and Therapeutic Communication in Mental Health Nursing

Medicines Management in Mental Health Nursing

Mental Health Law in Nursing

Physical Healthcare and Promotion in Mental Health Nursing

Promoting Recovery in Mental Health Nursing

Psychosocial Interventions in Mental Health Nursing

ADULT NURSING TITLES:

Acute and Critical Care in Adult Nursing (2nd Ed)

Caring for Older People in Nursing

Dementia Care in Nursing

Medicines Management in Adult Nursing

Nursing Adults with Long Term Conditions (2nd Ed)

Safeguarding Adults in Nursing Practice

You can find more information on each of these titles and our other learning resources at **www.sagepub.co.uk**. Many of these titles are also available in various e-book formats, please visit our website for more information.

About the authors

Daryl Evans was formerly an associate professor in nursing and health promotion at Middlesex University, where she was programme leader for the BSc top-up degree in Health Promotion. She is an experienced nurse and nurse teacher, and integrated health promotion practice into her role at the university. Her professional interests include empowerment of patients and settings-based health promotion.

Dina Coutsaftiki was formerly a senior lecturer at Middlesex University, where she taught health promotion on the BSc top-up degree in Health Promotion and on the BSc Nursing degree. Her research interests are in the field of health promotion with special focus on reproductive health.

Patricia Fathers was a senior lecturer at Middlesex University and taught on the BSc top-up degree in Health Promotion. She has taught health promotion to both nursing students and multidisciplinary healthcare students. This role has provided some insight into the needs of students as they engage in the study of health promotion.

Introduction

Who is this book for?

This book is written for students of nursing who are developing knowledge and skills in health promotion and public health. Although primarily aimed at students, it will also be useful for qualified nurses improving their practice and their role as mentors to students. Any health professionals undertaking health promotion in their practice may find aspects of the book helpful for reviewing what they do and planning improvements.

Health promotion and public health are essential components of the nurse's role. The knowledge and skills required may seem to be a vast volume of learning of a whole different subject in its own right. We intend this book to more directly apply what is relevant to nursing and, in particular, to help nursing students to understand how the subject specifically relates to them. The book will show how health promotion and public health are integral to any nurse's role, whether that is in community or hospital care, in the NHS or in the independent or charity sectors.

Third edition

This third edition has been generally updated and revised. Firstly, there have been changes relevant to nursing in that there is a new NMC Code, which we have referred to in suggestions for your portfolio compilation in Chapter 8. Then, in new NHS planning, there is the 5 Year Forward View that, among other things, highlights a failure to take prevention seriously, calls for a radical upgrade generally and re-emphasises the public health role of the nurse.

Secondly, the Government has created changes in public health policy to do with lifestyle choices. There are amendments and additions to policies and strategies concerning smoking, alcohol and healthy eating. Obesity in children has been re-addressed with a particular emphasis on sugar intake. More patient participation has been discussed in strategic planning for health screening, self-management and antibiotic awareness. All of which impacts on the role of the nurse in educating patients.

It has been a time of much change and also of much controversy about the changes. We hope to have made this third edition helpful to your learning and we also hope to excite your interest further in the political dimension to health promotion and public health.

Book structure

When we wrote the first edition we decided to take a less conventional approach to the chapters in the book, which we have kept for the second and third editions. Our experience in practising health promotion and public health in nursing, as well as in teaching nurses, has taught us that theories and principles need to be applied to the real world of nursing.

We start the book with a chapter on 'Thinking health promotion'. Nurses need to think about this subject first, before considering the whole of public health. To think as a promoter of health puts you into a set of ideas that are different from nursing, yet transferable into your practice. Instead of just defining health promotion, the chapter encourages you to see the international context and political dimensions of improving health. The chapter looks at theories informing health promotion and introduces two models of practice that are followed up in further chapters.

Chapter 2, 'Tackling lifestyle change', is where we address one of the biggest issues: persuading and enabling people to live healthily through making healthier choices. This goal can be difficult to achieve and take far longer than you expect. It is relevant to your work with individual patients and their families, and to your work with larger communities. Mostly nurses seem to think that it is just a case of giving more information, but the chapter illustrates that this may not be the answer. This chapter enables you to structure the way you give the best information, advice and support about making healthier lifestyle choices.

Chapter 3, 'Encouraging health screening', focuses on the nurse's role in promoting attendance to screening opportunities, as we feel there is not enough emphasis on this in nursing education. Many screening systems exist in the NHS but nurses often know little about them. It is clear to us that being able to talk to patients about the pros and cons of attending screening is essential, even if you are not working in a screening system yourself. You can be the resource the patient, family or members of the public use to find out what happens and whether they should attend.

Chapter 4 is about 'Teaching patients'. As it is fundamental to the nurse's role, the education of patients and their families is generally well understood and practised by nurses. We would argue, then, that practice still needs to improve. Too often the teaching a patient needs ends up as giving information at the point of discharge from hospital or is not done because nurses feel that there is not enough time. The chapter gives some practical ideas and encouragement to make teaching patients a more integrated part of your daily practice.

Chapter 5, 'Supporting self-management', is a topic of increasing importance to healthcare across the world, and is appearing more in the literature and policy setting of many countries. Health services must allocate more resources to enable the growing numbers of people living with long-term conditions to help themselves. In the interests of cost-effective healthcare and in the interests of empowerment of patients, nurses must develop the skills to support self-management. The chapter includes some ideas and systems many nurses are as yet unaware of. Focusing on the learned tendency to provide care, and on the learned tendency of patients to expect care, has made nurses less able to facilitate patients to become partners in their care.

The subject of Chapter 6, 'Considering public health', has been deliberately left until later in the book. Health promotion (as part of public health) is what nurses mostly do, but it is important to develop an awareness of the wider role. The term 'public health' is being increasingly used in literature and policy documents with the (correct) assumption that it includes health promotion, or what is often termed 'health improvement'. Even the general public is developing a greater awareness of what public health can achieve, through news items about outbreaks of communicable diseases and political debates about dealing with the so-called obesity epidemic and the increase in type 2 diabetes. The chapter gives you some idea of the functions of public health and of your role in addressing the wider determinants of health and consequences of unhealthy environments.

Chapter 7, 'Managing health promotion in practice', helps you to develop a more coordinating and managing role in improving health through nursing practice. It looks at the idea of people being in settings (places) where they work, live, learn and receive care. You will see the professional skills needed to continue developing public health and health promotion, including project planning and partnership working.

Chapter 8 is 'Keeping up your skills', and challenges you to plan to learn more and gain more skills. The chapter includes useful and practical ways to keep up to date with information and to plan your lifelong learning. It puts reflection, planning your learning and portfolio compilation into the context of your health promotion role.

Requirements for the NMC *Standards for Pre-registration Nursing Education* and the Essential Skills Clusters

The Nursing and Midwifery Council (NMC) has established standards of competence to be met by applicants to different parts of the register, and these are the standards it considers necessary for safe and effective practice in relation to health promotion and public health. In addition to the competencies, the NMC has set out specific skills that nursing students must be able to perform at various points of an education programme. These are known as Essential Skills Clusters (ESCs). This book is structured so that it will help you to understand and meet the competencies and ESCs required for entry to the NMC register. The relevant competencies and ESCs are presented at the start of each chapter so that you can clearly see which ones the chapter addresses. There are generic standards that all nursing students, irrespective of their field, must achieve, and field-specific standards relating to each field of nursing: mental health, children's, learning disability and adult nursing. This book includes the latest standards for 2010 onwards, taken from *Standards for Pre-registration Nursing Education* (NMC, 2010).

Learning features

Learning from reading text is not always easy. Therefore, to provide variety and to assist with the development of independent learning skills and the application of theory to practice, this book contains activities, case studies, scenarios, further reading, useful websites and other materials to enable you to participate in your own learning. You will need to develop your own study skills and 'learn how to learn' to get the best from the material. The book cannot provide all the answers, but instead provides a framework for your learning.

The activities in the book, in particular, will help you to make sense of, and learn about, the material being presented. Some activities ask you to reflect on aspects of practice, or your experience of it, or the people or situations you encounter. *Reflection* is an essential skill in nursing, and it helps you to understand the world around you and often to identify how things might be improved. Other activities will help you develop key graduate skills such as your ability to *think critically* about a topic in order to challenge received wisdom, or your ability to *research a topic and find appropriate information and evidence*, and to be able to *make decisions* using that evidence in situations that are often difficult and time-pressured. *Communication* and *working as part of a team* are core to all nursing practice, and some activities will ask you to carry out team-work activities or think about your communication skills to help develop these.

All the activities require you to take a break from reading the text, think through the issues presented and carry out some independent study, possibly using the internet. Where appropriate, there are outline answers presented at the end of each chapter, and these will help you to understand more fully your own reflections and independent study. Remember, academic study will always require independent work; attending lectures will never be enough to be successful on your programme, and these activities will help to deepen your knowledge and understanding of the issues under scrutiny and give you practice at working on your own.

You might want to think about completing these activities as part of your personal development plan (PDP) or portfolio. After completing the activity, write it up in your PDP or portfolio in a section devoted to that particular skill, then look back over time to see how far you have developed. You can also do more of the activities for a key skill that you have identified a weakness in, which will help your skill and confidence in this area.

There is a glossary of terms at the end of the book, which provides an interpretation of some key terminology in the context of the subject of the book. Glossary terms are in **bold** in the first instance that they appear.

All chapters have further reading and/or useful websites listed at the end, with notes to show you why we think they will be helpful to you.

We hope you enjoy this third edition of our book, and good luck with your studies.

Chapter 1
Thinking health promotion

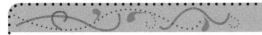

continued . . .

By the second progression point:

3. Understands the concept of public health and the benefits of healthy lifestyles and the potential risks involved with various lifestyles or behaviours, for example substance misuse, smoking, obesity.
4. Recognises indicators of unhealthy lifestyles.

By the third progression point:

18. Discusses sensitive issues in relation to public health and provides appropriate advice and guidance to individuals, communities and populations, for example contraception, substance misuse, smoking, obesity.

Chapter aims

By the end of this chapter you will be able to:

- define health and health promotion;
- discuss the contribution of the World Health Organization (WHO) to the development and practice of health promotion;
- appreciate the contribution of health promotion strategies to the promotion of good health and well-being;
- understand and integrate theories and models of health promotion into nursing practice.

Introduction

This chapter will encourage you to think about health promotion in relation to your nursing practice. Thinking like a health-promoting nurse will enable you to integrate the principles and practice of health promotion into your nursing care. How do you think like a health promoter? To do so, you need to view patients beyond their presenting medical diagnosis or condition and be mindful that you can contribute and support patients to improve their health by adopting an **empowering** approach while delivering care related to recovery from illness.

The chapter explores the concept of health and how this informs your health promotion practice. It enables you to develop your knowledge and understanding of the health promotion concept and its contribution to improving the health and quality of life of the individual and the population at large. The chapter explores the origin of health promotion and discusses international and national health strategies and their contribution to the development of your health promotion practice. Theories and models of health are examined in order to enable you to structure your health promotion practice.

What does it mean to be healthy?

··

Case study: What does it mean to be healthy?

Peter, a 52-year-old school teacher, underwent pancreatectomy and chemotherapy following a diagnosis of an advanced pancreatic cancer. As a result of removing his pancreas he is on insulin injections. He says:

'I have accepted my diagnosis and now I want to live a normal life. I am confident and competent in self-injecting the prescribed insulin. Shahita, my partner, is my rock. We are able to set realistic and achievable daily goals. Since my illness we have adopted a healthy lifestyle. Our diet, including the diet of Leon (our dog), is much healthier and also we are more physically active. I take Leon for a walk in the nearby park daily. I enjoy the fresh air and meeting the regular dog walkers.

I am back to full-time work. I enjoy teaching and I get a lot of personal satisfaction knowing that I contribute to my pupils' learning and development. I value the daily structure and social interaction offered by my work. I receive encouragement and support from my colleagues. We are able to have a laugh. However, I am aware that some colleagues feel that I am too ill to be working. They all know that my expected survival time is 18 months.

I have accepted that I do not have long to live; however, 18 months is still a long time. I still have inspirations and dreams. I want the remainder of my life to be lived in full. Shahita and I decided to get married and to have a huge wedding in three months' time. We have booked our holiday to Australia where we are planning to have our honeymoon. I feel that I am doing the things I always wanted to do but somehow I never got around to doing. I have made a will: I want to put my financial and private affairs into order before the inevitable happens.

Shahita and I talk a lot about death. I am not afraid of dying but I am afraid of how I will die. Will I be in pain? I am very lucky to live next door to Helen, a retired midwife and health visitor. I have known her all my life. She actually delivered me! I have frequent conversations with Helen, updating her with my medical progress, and I am able to seek her advice. She is able to explain things to me. I find her a great emotional support. I have very open and confidential conversations with Helen. I can shed a tear in front of Helen without feeling embarrassed or less of a man.

In the evenings I feel quite tired. I tend to spend most evenings reading, for example, the Bible *or one of the many novels I have in my library. I also watch television, mainly the daily news programmes as I like to keep abreast of the day's events. Some evenings my siblings will come to visit. I enjoy reminiscing with them about the past and the good old days. Overall I have good and bad days like everybody else.'*

··

The case study illustrates that different people have different views of what it means to be healthy. For example, some of Peter's work colleagues view health as being free from disease. Peter, on the other hand, is in remission and views health as personal fulfilment.

Exploring the concept of health

You need to develop a comprehensive understanding of the health concept because it informs and shapes your health promotion practice. One important point to bear in mind is that an individual's health status is not static. It is constantly changing throughout the day and is evolving throughout a lifetime. Have you noticed how you feel different at different times of the day – for example, in the morning you may have felt very energetic and by midday you may feel exhausted – or how your mood fluctuates during the day?

Health encompasses the following different dimensions.

- **Physical**: this is quite obvious as it relates to the functions of your body, for example, 'I am not well because I have a headache.'

- **Emotional**: this can relate to how you cope with feelings, such as anxiety and depression, or your ability to recognise your own emotions, such as fear and joy.

- **Intellectual**: this means that you have the ability to think clearly and coherently.

- **Sexual**: this means that you have the ability and freedom to establish intimate, loving relationships as well as the choice and ability to procreate.

- **Social**: this means that you have the ability to make and maintain relationships with other people, for example, having friends.

- **Spiritual**: this means that you are able to achieve peace of mind or are able to be at peace with your own self. As a nurse you must recognise that this is not only associated with religion. People who do not have a religion can achieve spiritual health by adopting principles of behaviour that lead to spirituality.

Activity 1.1 is designed to enable you to develop a clear understanding of the above health dimensions.

Activity 1.1	*Critical thinking*

Review Peter's case study above and discuss either with your peers or with a member of your family the following questions regarding Peter's health.

- Is he physically healthy?
- Is he emotionally healthy?
- Is he intellectually healthy?
- Is he sexually healthy?
- Is he socially healthy?
- Is he spiritually healthy?

Were there any differences of opinion? Were all of you able to support your argument?

An outline answer is provided at the end of the chapter.

Activity 1.1 has demonstrated to you that health is a very difficult concept to define. When you discussed Peter's health dimensions, what personal factors influenced your own assessment?

The meaning of health can be influenced by a multitude of factors, such as family and cultural background, religion, educational level, gender, ethnicity and **social class**. Outside influences include the effects of the media, social environment and government policies. In addition, the individual's personal life experience will influence his or her views of health.

These influences apply equally to **lay** people and health professionals. For example, if you reflect back from the start of your nursing studies up to the present time, you may realise that your past and current views about health are different. This can be attributed to the influence of your professional socialisation in the clinical practice and the nursing knowledge you have gained. As a result your health views have been reshaped as you have been exposed to a new professional culture and have developed new expertise.

Lay perceptions of health

As a nurse you are working in **partnership** with patients and their families, aiming to establish an interactive therapeutic relationship that encourages patients and families to participate in their care and to take responsibility for their health. Therefore, you need to give 'voice' and 'choice' to patients (DH, 2006a). To facilitate this process you have to seek out their health views. Knowing their health views enables you to design and implement health promotion programmes relevant to patients and communities.

Lay people's perspectives of health have been researched extensively over the last 50 years. Some people may view health:

- *in terms of not being ill* – 'I am well today because I do not have a cold or a headache';
- *in the context of physical fitness* – taking regular exercise and being fit;
- *in terms of control and risk* – binge drinking is seen as a health risk while being able to drink 'normal' amounts of alcohol is seen as being in control and having the ability to manage health;
- *in terms of not having a health problem that interferes with daily life* – an elderly person may consider being healthy as being able to walk or cook or going out to visit friends;
- *in the context of social relationships* – having friends and family around for social support and interaction;
- *as psychosocial well-being* – emotional well-being is being happy and undertaking recreational activities such as going on holidays.

As you can see, lay people's concept of health is diverse, ranging from the functional and medical perspective to the psychosocial perspective. The different views are associated with social class issues, for example working-class people may see health from the functional perspective while the higher **socio-economic status** groups may see health from the psychosocial perspective. Age and gender are contributing factors; young men may view health from the physical activity perspective, while women may emphasise the social perspective of having friends and family around them. You need to address these influences when you plan your health promotion practice (Chapters 4 and 7), aiming to deliver a personalised health promotion practice that empowers patients to improve their health status.

How do health professionals view the concept of health? Are there any differences between lay and professional views?

Professional perceptions of health

Health professionals view the concept in relation to the following health models. Understanding the different models of health will enable you to understand how the different health professionals with whom you work interpret health and working in partnership (see Chapter 7), to help you to develop a health promotion practice with common goals and objectives to improve patients' health.

Medical model

Under the medical model of health your practice has a disease orientation instead of a positive health orientation. You view patients only in terms of their presenting illnesses, therefore you focus on the physical dimension of health without taking into consideration the other dimensions previously discussed in this chapter. This means that you view each patient as a body (which includes brain function) in terms of possible defective parts and your aim is to repair the parts. It means that you manage the medical diagnosis of patients. Your health promotion will focus on teaching/coaching patients, on giving them information regarding their treatment and ensuring that they will understand the pathophysiology of the medical condition or disease concerned. You will be involved, for example, in teaching and demonstrating to patients such things as how to use their inhalers to improve their breathing without considering other factors that may influence recovery, such as personal circumstances and health inequalities.

The medical model of health can be criticised for having an authoritarian approach to patient care. The patient is seen as a passive participant. All decisions are made by the professionals 'who know best'. It encourages patients' dependency on doctors and nurses. However, you need to recognise the valuable and significant contribution of biomedical factors to health improvement in the arena of public health.

In summary, from the health promotion and public health perspective (Chapter 6), the main focus in the medical model is on treatment and cure. It provides the basis for encouraging patients' **concordance** with current treatment and also enables you to use this as a building-block when you are considering self-management strategies (Chapter 5).

Holistic model

A well-documented and widely used definition of health by many health professionals is that of the World Health Organization (WHO, 1948): *Health is a state of complete physical, mental and social wellbeing and not merely the absence of disease.* The combination of physical, social and mental well-being is known as the 'health triangle'.

The model expands on the medical model of health by embracing the concept of well-being. However, the definition implies a utopian view of achievement of health. It is therefore, arguably, idealistic in that it is impossible to attain a 'complete state' of health. One may also argue that it excludes people such as Peter (who has a terminal illness), or people with chronic diseases (for example, schizophrenia, Parkinson's) or a disability (for example, visual impairment or learning disabilities), or people who, due to circumstances beyond their control, such as poverty, are unable to achieve optimum health.

In health promotion terms the **holistic** approach emphasises the need to integrate health education and prevention activities that constitute evidence-based practice. Your practice has to be informed not only by the medical aspects of health but also by local and national health strategies. The model encourages a reorientation of NHS provision from the acute health **sector** to primary care (community health sector).

Wellness model

The WHO, moving with social trends and political ideologies, furthered the concept of health by developing a wellness model, which is built on the principles of the holistic model.

The Ottawa Charter for health promotion considered health to be not just a 'state', but a *resource for everyday life, not the objective of living. It is a positive concept emphasising social and personal resources, as well as physical capabilities* (WHO, 1986). This definition is relevant to current health promotion practice, which strives to improve quality of life of all people regardless of their health status. It includes healthy people, people with disabilities, people with mental health issues, people with learning disabilities and people with long-term conditions. It highlights the need for the individual to be resilient by adapting to life changes such as illnesses and changes in socio-economic circumstances.

The model encourages health professionals to promote **anti-discriminatory** practice. For example, you as a health promoter, through the application of an empowering approach to your practice (Chapter 5), will support people with physical impairment, such as wheelchair users, to manage their condition effectively and lead independent lives. You will act as an enabler to facilitate them to adapt positively to life's changes and to strive for personal growth and fulfilment by developing problem-solving skills and increasing their **self-esteem**. The model encourages patients' active participation in the decision-making process by encouraging them to value their own expertise and experience.

Thinking about the complexities of health through the different perspectives of the three models discussed above could be confusing. We suggest that you consider the WHO (1948) definition of health in combination with its 1986 definition as a resource.

In this way nurses can act in partnership with other healthcare professionals, patients and their families, to devise an eclectic model of health incorporating the three components of body (physical), mind (mental) and community (social) aspects of health, as well as the ability of people to gain control of their own health (adapting and growing). To assist you we will be looking in future chapters at:

- enabling patients to change their health behaviours (Chapter 2);
- empowering them to understand their illnesses (Chapter 4);
- supporting them to 'self-manage' their illnesses (Chapter 5).

However, before you develop your nursing practice to integrate health promotion principles, you need to have a deeper understanding of the health promotion concept.

Defining health promotion

Health promotion is about improving the health status of individuals and the population as a whole. Key to the term 'health promotion' is the word 'promotion'. This means placing the notion of the absence of disease and well-being at the forefront of your nursing practice. This shift in emphasis will help you think about improving, advancing, encouraging and supporting your patients to achieve optimum health. These activities are all part of a health-promoting perspective.

Today health promotion is an important focus of UK public policy in all sectors, with an emphasis on the social and environmental aspects as much as the physical and mental-health perspectives. Therefore, nurses have to view health promotion from both a holistic and a wellness model of health. It is helpful to understand the major socio-economic determinants of health. Very often these are outside the control of the individual, but they can have an enormous effect on the individual's health; for example, employment redundancy may lead to poverty and may affect the individual's physical and mental health by, for example, increasing the chances of developing coronary heart disease or depression.

The fundamental aim of health promotion is to empower an individual or a community to take control of aspects of their lives that have a detrimental effect on their health. The WHO (1986) defines health promotion as *a process of enabling people to increase control over, and to improve, their health*. This definition implies that you need to act as an enabler by strengthening knowledge, attitudes, skills and capabilities of your patients to overcome negative health. Additionally, governments are urged by the WHO to formulate health strategies to facilitate this enabling process.

Activity 1.2 aims to encourage you to explore the scope of health promotion by considering a selection of possible health-promoting activities.

Activity 1.2   *Critical thinking*

Which of the following activities do you consider to be health-promoting by enabling or empowering?

- A TV advertisement around the Christmas period that encourages the public 'not to drink and drive'.
- A radio message on your local radio encouraging young people to ring a helpline if they feel that they are victims of abuse.
- Practice nurses delivering a smoking cessation programme.

---

continued . . .

- Nurses teaching carers how to feed their loved one at home via a PEG (percutaneous endoscopic gastrostomy) feeding tube.
- Legislation on the compulsory use of car seat belts.
- The Alcohol Health Alliance, representing all major medical and nursing organisations, **lobbying** the government to increase the minimum price for alcoholic drinks.
- Local authorities organising park walks for young mothers.
- Health agencies such as Age UK giving information during winter on how to keep warm.
- Environmental health officers inspecting restaurants and cafés to monitor hygiene standards.
- Restaurants providing food information on their menus such as the fat content of their lamb moussaka.
- Practice nurses immunising older people against the flu virus.
- Nurses washing their hands.
- Student nurses receiving training on moving and handling.
- Supporting people with learning disabilities to use public transport.

An outline answer is provided at the end of the chapter.

Health promotion encompasses a very broad range of activities that aim to facilitate people to achieve a full and healthy life, which is based on the broader view of health. Nowadays, the emphasis is on acting on the socio-environmental, as well as physical, influences of health. Thus, there is a need for a variety of professionals (i.e., not only healthcare professionals), organisations and government departments to work together to promote health in all sorts of ways, as indicated in Activity 1.2 and as you will see in the next section. This modern view of the potential for improving health began in the 1980s with an international shift in emphasis to give this broader range.

The origin of health promotion

Health promotion gained momentum in the global **health agenda** in the later part of the twentieth century. This took place against a backdrop of discontent and frustration in international political and public opinion with the status quo of the medically dominated healthcare systems. Those systems were failing to combat ill health and to meet the health needs of the populations they were serving, despite a constant increase in financial investment.

Health promotion emerged as a process to shift healthcare provision away from a hospital setting centred on the medicalisation of health towards a community setting informed by the principles of public health (Chapter 6). This transition was facilitated as the holistic and wellness models of health started to gain momentum and the dominant medical model started to be eroded.

The WHO has been instrumental in the development of health promotion. Its commitment to using health promotion to improve global health is seen in a number of international charters and declarations. The most significant are the Ottawa Charter, the Adelaide Conference and the Bangkok Charter.

Concept summary: The Ottawa Charter

This charter (WHO, 1986) created the following principles for health promotion action, which are still relevant today.

Build healthy public policy

Health promotion goes beyond healthcare. **Policy** makers across all government sectors must consider health consequences and accept responsibility for health. This means that, when considering transport, housing or employment policies at local or national level, they should be asking about their health implications. In addition, central governments should make policy decisions that improve health such as, for example, the smoking ban and wearing car seat belts.

The key issue in achieving a successful health promotion policy is joint action between the different sectors at a national level and interprofessional working at a local level. All of the diverse parties involved in policy making have to ensure that these policies enable all people to make healthier choices.

Create supportive environments

The environment we live in affects our health; for example, changing patterns of life, work and leisure and our natural environment have a significant impact on our health. Therefore, health promotion has to influence the generation of living and working conditions that are safe, stimulating, satisfying and enjoyable (Chapter 7).

Strengthen community action

Health promotion works through concrete and effective community action in setting priorities, making decisions, and planning and implementing them to achieve better health. At the heart of this process is community empowerment (Chapter 7).

Develop personal skills

Health promotion supports personal and social development through the provision of information, education or health-enhancing **life skills**. It has to enable people to learn, throughout life, to prepare themselves for all their health-related problems and to cope with long-term conditions and injuries (Chapters 4 and 5).

Reorient health services

The role of the health sector must move beyond its traditional responsibility for providing curative and clinical health. In the UK the NHS should focus more on the prevention of illness and the promotion of positive wellness.

Reorientation also involves changes being made to professional education in order to meet the health needs of the population. This can be seen in the current changes taking place in nurse education, which has moved to a graduate level – a change that aims to prepare nurses to be appropriately qualified and equipped to meet and serve the health needs of people in the twenty-first century.

The Ottawa Charter remains one of the most influential charters within the field of health promotion and public health. It is based on a **strategy** of enabling people to control health, advocating that health must be prioritised in all sectors and mediating between possible partners to improve health.

Following on from Ottawa, the Adelaide Conference (WHO, 1988) brought health promotion practice to new levels with health being viewed as a 'human right'. Health was no longer to be seen as a mere commodity. The conference introduced the concept of **equity**, highlighting that all people and patients have to be treated the same.

Later, the Bangkok Charter (WHO, 2005) urged all global governments to integrate effective health promotion interventions into their domestic and foreign policies. They are asked to implement interventions that have been proven to contribute to positive health and well-being into everything they do, whether it is town planning, road expansion or financial cutbacks. Policies, not only in times of peace but also in times of war and conflict, need to be 'healthy', so, for example, nurses who are working in the armed forces in war zones such as Iraq, Afghanistan and Syria have to use a repertoire of evidence-based health interventions to promote a sense of well-being in the soldiers.

The WHO, in addition to international charters and declarations, has placed health promotion at the heart of its current global health agenda by its *Health-for-All Policy for the Twenty-first Century* (World Health Assembly, 1998), by continuing the previous vision of the *Health for All by the Year 2000* strategy (WHO, 1981).

Concept summary: *WHO Health-for-All Policy for the Twenty-first Century*

The *Health for All* (HFA) policy calls for social justice, which means that each person should be treated fairly and equitably. It lists ten global health targets set out in three domains, reflecting the most prevalent health problems in the world.

Improving health outcomes

- Health equity: this will be assessed by measuring a child's growth, i.e. height and weight levels for age (children under five years).
- Survival: to improve maternal mortality rates, child mortality rates (under five years) and life expectancy.
- Reverse global trends of five major pandemics (TB, malaria, HIV/AIDS, tobacco-related diseases and violence/trauma) by implementing disease control programmes.
- Eradicate and eliminate certain diseases (measles, leprosy and vitamin A and iodine deficiencies).

Determinants of health

- Improve access to water, sanitation, food and shelter.
- Measures to enhance healthy lifestyles and weaken damaging ones.

(Continued)

(Continued)

Health policies

- Develop, implement and monitor national HFA policies.
- Improve access to comprehensive, essential quality healthcare.
- Implement global and national health information and surveillance systems.
- Support research for health.

Each region of the WHO (Africa, Americas, Southeast Asia, Europe, Eastern Mediterranean and Western Pacific) and subsequently individual countries have modified and incorporated this strategy into their own plans to meet the health needs of the populations they serve. The WHO (1998) developed a strategy for Europe known as Health 21. The following case study outlines the different global health challenges.

Case study: Different global health challenges

Mrs Shah, a registered nurse, has returned to England after spending two years working as a volunteer nurse in one of Africa's underdeveloped countries. She gives a seminar to her work colleagues, aiming to share her working experience in Africa.

Her account supports the need for a global health strategy and highlights the importance of gaining the political commitment of international organisations, as well as national governments, to implement the WHO's strategy. In summary, Nurse Shah highlighted the following issues:

'Every day, people of all ages in sub-Saharan Africa die unnecessarily. The main cause is infectious diseases such as malaria, tuberculosis, HIV/AIDS and diarrhoea. One of the biggest challenges healthcare providers face is the delivery of adequate healthcare for people living with chronic lifestyle conditions. People in rural areas have to walk many miles to access care. Many die in transit.

Another frustrating thing for me was the fact that healthcare professionals work in isolation, particularly those working in rural settings, and they could not keep abreast of the latest information on epidemics. This also precludes them from sharing their information with the global health community. Nurses in the region are increasingly faced with the burden of providing healthcare to rural populations, much more than the doctors. Enhancing health professionals', especially nurses', access to relevant accurate and up-to-date clinical information is vital to improving healthcare.'

Recognising aspects of the international view of health promotion will help you to understand the global background and how this influences the UK's health agenda. As a member state of WHO (European Region) and the European Union (at the time of writing) the UK is instrumental in helping to formulate international strategies and in making decisions as to how to implement those strategies at a regional level within the European Union countries and also at a national (UK) level.

UK national strategic policies for public health and health promotion

In the UK the concept of health promotion can be traced as far back as the nineteenth century, forming part of the public health movement for sanitary reforms to improve the ill health of people living in overcrowded industrial towns. Florence Nightingale embraced the principles of public health to inform nursing practice (Nightingale, 1859).

The first ever public health strategy published in the UK was *The Health of the Nation* (DH, 1992) by the then Conservative government. It has to be commended for responding to the call for 'health for all by the year 2000' by the World Health Organization (WHO, 1981). It provides an example of an effort being made at a policy level to improve health by encompassing both prevention and health promotion. However, it could be criticised for adopting a medical approach (that is, by aiming to prevent premature death due to ill health) to the detriment of addressing the broader economic and social factors that influence health.

This was superseded by the strategies of the new Labour government in *Saving Lives: Our Healthier Nation* (DH, 1999) and, later, *Choosing Health: Making Healthier Choices Easier Choices* (DH, 2004b). The former set targets to be achieved by 2010, continuing the theme set by its predecessor to tackle ill health. It also took into consideration health inequalities (Acheson, 1998) by addressing **social exclusion**. The strategy embraced a social model of health by promoting collaboration between health and local authorities. The latter strategy goes further by recognising the social, environmental, economic and cultural impacts on health. However, there was an absence of national policies (social and economic) to tackle the fundamental causes of inequality. The focus was on lifestyle issues aiming to change individual behaviour, thus introducing the notion of **victim blaming**. Scotland, Wales and Northern Ireland had their own similar strategies.

All these health strategies use health promotion to facilitate the achievement of **health improvement** and to encourage people to 'make healthy choices easier choices', political jargon originated by the WHO and used to achieve **health gain**. The policies aim to improve the health of the individual and the population by addressing the wider issues that affect health, such as health inequalities and environmental issues.

The UK coalition government (2010 – 2015) produced its own strategy, *Healthy Lives, Healthy People: Our Strategy for Public Health in England* (DH, 2010b), which is still relevant at the time of writing (2016). It focuses on behaviour-change strategies that encourage individuals to engage in healthy behaviour and to take more control and responsibility for their own health, thereby moving away from the notion of the 'nanny state', whereby people expect the state to take care of their own health (Chapters 2 and 6). Scotland, Wales and Northern Ireland constructed their own strategies based on that of England.

As the various successive governments endeavour to improve people's health and to promote positive health, healthcare professionals have witnessed the establishment of the following.

- **NHS Direct:** launched in 1998 as a nurse-led telephone helpline and internet service providing information and advice on health to the public. The coalition government phased out NHS Direct. In April 2013 the NHS 111 free-of-charge service was launched. It operates 365 days a year, aiming to improve access to the NHS when patients are in need of medical help or advice, but in circumstances where the need is not urgent enough to justify making a 999 call. It is staffed by fully trained advisers supported by nurses and paramedics. It is driven by the ideology to manage patients in a more cost-effective and integrated way. Its launch has already been controversial. Healthcare professionals and patients have criticised the system as being a 'cut-price' replacement of NHS Direct nurses, with telephone advisers lacking professional training in healthcare, thereby leading to delays in treatment and putting patients' lives at risk. Since its launch the non-emergency 111 hotline has attracted a plethora of adverse publicity regarding its performance. Examples of such criticisms are:

  o Callers have complained about delays in their call been answered;

  o Callers have been asked inappropriate questions such as 'are you conscious?'. This is due to the fact that call handlers have to follow and adhere to an automated computerised questionnaire system leaving callers feeling vulnerable, patronised and very frustrated. The automate computer system questionnaire has also contributed to clogging up the accident and emergency departments by sending patients to those departments unnecessarily.

However the 111 service does provide a valuable service to the public, as it provides a single point of contact whereby patients or their carers can get urgent help and advice regarding their health problem as presented at the time of the call.

- **NICE (National Institute for Health and Care Excellence):** responsible for providing national guidance on promoting good health, and preventing and treating ill health.

- **Public health observatories:** established in 2000 in each NHS region. Their role is to ensure that health and social care systems are equipped with health intelligence to improve health and reduce inequalities, to promote research and to set up disease registers.

- **Health Protection Agency (HPA):** set up in 2003 to protect the public from infectious diseases and environmental hazards. The HPA is one of a number of quangos (quasi-autonomous non-governmental organisations) that were abolished on 1 April 2013. This protection function was transferred to central NHS control.

- **Patient Advice and Liaison Services (PALS):** designed to bring citizens more closely into decision-making processes.

- **Expert Patients Programme (EPP):** to help people manage their own illnesses (see Chapter 5, pages 101-3).

- **NHS walk-in centres:** launched in 1999, aiming to provide the general public with more convenient access to NHS services matching modern living patterns, and managed by local community health organisations to deal with minor illnesses and injuries. They are predominantly nurse-led. As from April 2013 such centres have been financed by the area's Clinical Commissioning Groups.

- **Polyclinics** (more recently called multi-centres): established on the recommendations of Lord Darzi (a parliamentary undersecretary in the House of Lords), they are a network of GPs in multi-purpose health centres, which provide some hospital services such as X-rays, minor surgery and outpatients' treatment.

As well as these strategic innovations, we have seen a focus on addressing **inequalities in health**, which has been informed by WHO's work (see Chapter 6 for a fuller explanation).

We now go on to look at health promotion theories and models to guide your work. We previously looked at theories of health; however, theory is also important in 'thinking health promotion', as without it we may act randomly and without the evidence to support practice. Theoretical structures are based on ideas from philosophical or organisational constructs and, more recently, are deduced from practice itself. You will find health promotion theories used throughout this book; here we give an overview of the most important ones. A model, as compared with a theory, is a framework that derives from theory and attempts to represent reality, rather like a model of a building representing the building's parts and functions. Models provide a systematic, well-researched approach to health promotion practice.

Theories informing health promotion

As with nursing, there are a number of theories that underpin the practice of health promotion. These are informed by a multitude of academic disciplines such as **epidemiology** and **demography**, ethics and law, health psychology and politics.

Epidemiology and demography

These disciplines provide information about a population's health status. The information focuses on the severity, range, frequency and duration of diseases, and the associated social disability and mortality. They also inform you about the relationship between ill-health and socio-demographic variables such as age, culture, economic status, educational attainment, employment status and ethnicity, including the geographical variable (north–south divide). They enable you to identify priorities, set targets (Chapters 4 and 7), plan and implement health promotion interventions suitable for a target group based on an assessment of its health needs and, finally, to evaluate their efficacy. For example, if the locality where you are working has a large older population with a high incidence of falls at home, you need to deliver health promotion programmes that enable them to avoid falls at home. Another example is organising child immunisation programmes if the locality has many families with young children.

Within the field of mental health, epidemiology and demography will enable you to ascertain the complexities of mental health and to deliver appropriate services to improve the health and social function of individuals suffering with mental illness. This can be achieved by providing local services for early detection, care, treatment and rehabilitation. Engagement in community health education programmes, in order to tackle the social stigma, myths and misconceptions surrounding mental health, is setting the ground for resettling people with mental illness back into the community, thereby safeguarding their human rights and dignity.

Modern epidemiology is shifting from a population level (traditional epidemiology), which was informed by a public health model taking into consideration the cultural and historical perspective of diseases, to an individual level informed by a model of science (tissues, cells, and anatomy and physiology). This has implications for health promotion policy as the focus will be on targeting solely the **pathophysiology** of disease to the exclusion of addressing and tackling the social determinants and their impact on health. Prevention will focus on behaviour change with the inherent notion of victim blaming.

In summary, epidemiology and demography together provide you with a scientific basis to determine the distribution and determinants of health and disease of the population you serve, and to determine the scope for health promotion practice.

Ethics and law

Ethics and law are concerned with making a series of value judgements about what health means to the individual or to the community and about whether, when and how to intervene. A central ethical question for you is what is acceptable or unacceptable. Ethics and law enable you to consider principles such autonomy, respect for the individual, freedom to make decisions without coercion, voluntary participation, confidentiality, informed consent, social justice, equity and the mental capacity of patients. These principles inform you how to develop a non-discriminatory and **non-judgemental** practice. You need to ensure that the patient is changing behaviour on a voluntary basis and by exercising free will. For example, if a smoker decides to continue smoking, after receiving health education on the risks of smoking and the accessibility and availability of smoking cessation programmes, you have to accept that he or she is exercising free will and choice without blaming him or her for failure to conform, known as victim blaming.

Your practice can be informed by the principles of *beneficence* and *non-maleficence*. These mean that your health promotion interventions promote good and also prevent, remove and avoid harm to your patients. These principles place the common (majority) good before individual considerations. An example is fluoridisation of drinking water supplies to promote dental health. This is beneficial to the majority even though it may not further benefit a minority.

You will be engaging in a diversity of health promotion practices across the different fields of nursing (Adult, Mental Health, Child and Learning Disabilities). Each field imposes a variety of ethical dilemmas. You will need to address these by using a collaborative approach (involving patients, families, doctors and other health professionals) and critically appraising your health promotion interventions using available evidence to consider the following questions.

- Does this health promotion practice impinge on the freedom or autonomy of the patients, for example implementation of a 'non-smoking policy' in a long-stay mental health unit?
- Is this health promotion intervention a source of collective good or benefit for patients, for example the provision of immunisation services for young children, bearing in mind the well-publicised controversy over MMR (measles, mumps and rubella) immunisation and its current health implications, or the screening for Down's syndrome during pregnancy?

- Does this health promotion practice encourage victim blaming and stigmatisation, for example health education focusing on lifestyle?

- Are the benefits of this health promotion provision equally distributed among all the people living in the area, for example access to health services for screening by people with learning disabilities, available resources in different languages, and policy setting that acknowledges different rules of faith?

- Does this health promotion practice safeguard confidentiality, dignity and mental capacity, for example in the cases of contraception and teenagers, or contraception and people with learning disabilities?

In summary, ethics and law inform your health promotion practice by ensuring that people should be free to achieve well-being. They must have real opportunities to live and act in accordance with their values and capabilities, and their participation must be voluntary.

Health psychology

Health psychology is a subdivision of psychology that seeks to explain how people behave in relation to their health. In promoting health we are interested in how people change to healthy behaviours. There are many individual theories to explain this, briefly explained below.

Theories of reasoned action and planned behaviour

These theories (Ajzen and Fishbein, 1980) increase understanding of the factors that influence people's intention to behave in a certain way, which in turn enables you to develop interventions that meet individuals' needs, for example the use of **peer education**. These theories do not explain the impact that emotions and religious beliefs have on behaviour, for example religious beliefs may contribute to stigmatisation of certain diseases such as HIV/AIDS.

The health belief model

This model (Becker, 1974) demonstrates that behaviour change is dependent upon the individual's belief about his or her susceptibility to a disease, severity of the illness, and the cost and benefit analysis involved in any change of behaviour. Becker's health belief model enables you to understand and predict why individuals will or will not participate in different prevention activities such as health screening programmes. Therefore, the model is useful in planning preventative services. However, it has very limited value in planning health promotion interventions to tackle addictive behaviours such as drug addiction because there is a lack of information on how to modify complex health beliefs associated with long-term and socially determined behaviours.

The health locus of control theory

This theory (Rotter, 1966) explains the extent to which people feel that they have control over events and how their personalities are shaped as a result of these beliefs. The theory suggests that people who feel in control of their lives (**internal locus of control**) are more likely to change their behaviour than people who feel powerless (**external locus of control**). This theory contributes to our understanding of people's engagement in the process of behaviour change. However, it lacks reliability as it is very difficult to predict behaviour on the grounds of attitude alone without taking into account the interaction between people and their environment.

The social cognitive theory

This theory (Bandura, 1977) provides a framework for understanding, predicting and changing behaviour. Bandura explored the concept of **self-efficacy**, or the belief an individual has in her or his ability to change or overcome difficulties. He claimed that human behaviour change is governed by the following principles:

- **self-efficacy**: an individual's confidence to carry out a certain behaviour;
- **expectancy**: the belief that a certain action will result in the desired outcome;
- **incentives**: where behaviour is guided by the value the individual places on the perceived outcome.

This will vary with different situations; for example, a smoker may be confident that he or she can resist smoking when other people smoke at work, but may be less confident that he or she can do this when in the pub socialising with smoker friends. This theory provides a powerful link between the individual, the environment and behaviour. However, the challenge is around the development of self-efficacy skills.

Overall, health psychology theories provide you with a sound understanding of human behaviour based on attitudes, beliefs, values, power and control, which can be used to help people change from risky behaviour and to adopt healthy behaviour by making healthier choices. However, reliance solely on behaviour change is restrictive and has been criticised as 'victim blaming' for placing the onus of change solely on the individual.

All these theories from other disciplines inform health promotion theory construction, just as theories from psychology, sociology, ethics and medicine all inform nursing theory. The next section looks at two models developed for planning health promotion initiatives: the first is a strategic planning model for community health promotion and the second is a model for encouraging behaviour change in individuals and groups.

Health promotion models

There is a variety of models that are informed by different theoretical perspectives such as health psychology; most acknowledge the need to improve health through education, prevention of illness, and promotion of positive wellness. Some models emphasise one aspect or another, but most can be adapted to incorporate thinking about the broader aspects of health improvement and address the Ottawa Charter principles and inequalities in health (Marmot, 2010).

Tannahill's (1985) model gives an overview of the three main organisational aspects of health promotion (see Chapter 2 for further explanation). It presupposes that health education has existed for many years, in schools for children and, for adults, mainly through health professionals and the media. It acknowledges the historical and current importance of preventive services in public health, such as immunisation and screening. In addition, following the WHO imperative to generate healthy policies, the model incorporates policy making as its third part. Overall, this model can be seen as a very useful planning, implementing and evaluating device for health promotion practice – educating about smoking, screening for smoking-related diseases and setting no-smoking policies. You can use this model as a thinking tool to imagine the whole of what you can set up as you plan health promotion for one patient, for groups of patients or for communities. According to Tannahill:

- *Health education* aims to facilitate positive health by increasing peoples' knowledge and therefore changing their beliefs, attitudes, values and behaviour leading to a positive health outcome.

- *Health protection* aims to promote positive health and the enhancement of well-being by the introduction of fiscal controls and the implementation of legislative action. For example, increased taxation on cigarettes facilitates the cessation of smoking; the introduction of the national living wage (HM Government, 2016a) reduces inequalities. Other examples include the 2012 Health and Social Care Act (DH, 2012a) that introduced a radical reorganisation of the health services in order to meet the needs of the population in the twenty-first century. Another legislative example is food labelling by introducing the inclusion of physical activity alongside calorie content on food packaging to combat obesity (NHS Choices, 2016).

- *Disease prevention* aims to reduce risks of ill health and to minimise the consequences of diseases. Traditionally, it can be categorised into three different levels. This is useful for thinking of the scope of preventive services and strategies.

  o *Primary prevention* targets healthy people and aims to empower them to continue their healthy status, for example by the uptake of flu vaccination. As a nurse you will be involved in activities that aim to reduce/minimise the incidences of illness in your serving population.

  o *Secondary prevention* targets people who are at risk of developing ill health, aiming to persuade them to seek screening such as, for example, cervical screening. Your aim is early detection. As a nurse operating in a clinical environment you are already involved in early detection by, for example, carrying out clinical activities such as urinalysis to detect diabetes.

  o *Tertiary prevention* targets unhealthy people, aiming to empower them through self-management of their illnesses by, for example, complying with medication. During the course of your nursing studies you will have participated in rehabilitation programmes designed to help patients regain their independence and return to normal life, for example after suffering a cardio-vascular accident.

The above classification of prevention enables you to address a variety of health issues, ranging from physical health problems and mental health to disability, across the different stages of people's life span and to design appropriate health promotion interventions. There is an enormous potential for nurses to play a more proactive role in the prevention of ill health by engaging in evidence-based activities as opposed to simply providing information and advice. Examples of good practice can be seen in smoking cessation programmes whereby personal counselling, pharmaceutical interventions and interprofessional working contribute to a successful outcome. Tannahill (2009) revised his original model to encompass a more holistic approach to health and to minimise the medicalisation of health by incorporating the following health-influencing aspects into the model's original three areas of activities:

- *Environmental, socio-economic and cultural factors* (see Chapter 7): environmental factors include the whole spectrum of structures that contribute to health, for example people's occupations, provision of recreational activities, health services and religion, all of which play a vital role in people's health and health behaviour;

- *Education and learning:* this is an important aspect as it enables you to acknowledge that people are individuals and have very personal educational needs as well as styles of learning when planning and devising your teaching programme (see Chapter 4);

- *Equity and diversity:* both these aspects are an integral part of your everyday nursing practice. As a nurse working in a multicultural and diverse society you are involved in promoting equal opportunities and fairness of care and treatment to all patients by respecting their diversity and responding to their health needs;

- *Community-led and community-based health promotion activity:* these aim to enable communities to take control of decisions relating to health issues as they are identified and determined by the population and not by the professionals.

Tannahill's revised model advocates health promotion interventions that promote empowerment by involving people in the decision-making process and in the development of life skills.

In summary, Tannahill's model provides a structured approach for organising, delivering and evaluating health promotion. Nurses can draw on practical experience to distil the model as health education, prevention and health policy form an integral part of nursing practice. It does not, however, inform you about what motivates individuals to change behaviour or how to sustain this change. It could be argued that it has a paternalistic approach to health promotion practice. The revised model considers the wider influences of health and it enables health promotors to use an empowering approach to their health promotion practice.

Prochaska and DiClemente's (1982) model is one that incorporates many aspects of health psychology (see Chapter 2 for further explanation). This model was developed to explain how individuals move towards adopting behaviour that will maintain good health. It uses stages of change as its core construct and integrates processes and principles of change derived from different theories, hence it is called 'transtheoretical'. The model presumes the individual will go through stages of changing health behaviour that are cyclical and shows that, having completed one change, the person may well go on to feel that she or he can make another.

Its main focus is on the individual's readiness to change or attempt to change towards a healthy behaviour. The key concepts of this model are: pre-contemplation, contemplation, decision and determination, action and maintenance.

- At first the individual does not think of making a change – 'I'm OK as I am' – perhaps influenced by health belief and attribution theory.

- Then something may happen to make her or him consider a change – 'Maybe I should do something about it.' The influence here could be what others say (social cognitive theory).

- Having made a tentative decision, the individual then wonders how to make the change – 'I'll look into it.' The internal locus of control is becoming stronger.

- The individual engages in a new behaviour, trying it out.

- Sustaining the change over time takes inner strength. Social support and self-efficacy help with this stage.

- At any time in the cycle, the individual may revert to unhealthy behaviour, known as a 'relapse stage'. It is important to acknowledge the individual's effort and achievements so far and instil in her or him a sense of self-worth for accomplished achievement during the process of change.

Many practitioners within the field of health promotion have supported the Prochaska and DiClemente (1982) model as it allows the practitioner to tailor interventions according to individuals' specific needs. However, you need to be aware that implementation of these interventions may be time-consuming, expensive and complicated. Therefore, the model's use may not be suitable in a very busy acute clinical setting, where patients stay for a short period of time and require rapid treatment, unless the aim of the encounter is refocused on just moving the patient from one stage to another. It will be appropriate for use in clinical areas such as mental health or in a community setting where rapid behaviour change is not necessary.

In summary, this model is useful from a programme planning perspective, as it enables you to plan health promotion activities that will influence behaviour change according to patients' stage of change and motivation to change. Examples will be the use of written material, use of media, organisation of health and/or social support events, providing personal counselling and follow-up consultations, aiming to raise awareness of a behaviour's risk and benefits, and providing support to facilitate change. Health psychology and health promotion models may explain some aspects of behaviour, but do not expect them to solve the problem! You have to be discerning with regard to your choice of model by being eclectic and flexible in your mode of approach, by being able to move from a bottom-up to a top-down approach according to the situation and problem.

There are other models and theories of health promotion and public health to be found in the literature. We have chosen to focus on these two examples, but encourage you to read around the subject and to think about which model or theory is being used when you read about health promotion initiatives (see Further reading at the end of this chapter).

Activity 1.3   *Reflection*

You are working as a registered nurse in a community-based health centre located in a diverse social and cultural setting. You have been designated as the lead nurse to design a health promotion programme for overweight young adults. Obesity has been identified by the annual local health report as a major health problem. You believe that a community-based health promotion programme that involves the locality's young adults in the planning of the programme will be more beneficial. You are of the opinion that their involvement will promote ownership and engagement. The programme will be funded by the local clinical commissioning group in partnership with the local authority.

Reflecting on this chapter's content, what theories/models will inform the programme's health promotion interventions?

An outline answer is provided at the end of the chapter

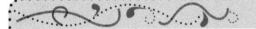

Chapter summary

This chapter has enabled you to develop an understanding of the health promotion concept, its origin and development in the UK up to the present day. It has explained how the perceived concept of health by patients and health professionals can influence health outcomes. The WHO views health promotion as instrumental in achieving global health and has identified nurses as key players who, working in partnership with others, can have a positive impact on health improvement. The WHO states that nurses can achieve this by acting as patients' advocates, mediators and enablers.

The promotion of positive health is the mutual responsibility of the individual, who has to take responsibility for his or her own health by adopting healthy behaviour, and of the state, which also has responsibility through the development and implementation of national and local health policies to address the wider determinants of health in order to improve the health status of the nation.

The chapter has examined different health promotion theories and models that enable you, as a nurse, to plan and implement health promotion within your nursing practice in order to empower patients to achieve optimum health.

Activities: brief outline answers

Activity 1.1: Critical thinking (page 8)

- **Physical**: No, Peter is not physically healthy as he has cancer and diabetes. However, according to Peter, he is physically healthy as he feels well and he is in remission. He is able to walk and go to work.

- **Emotional**: Yes, he has the ability to recognise his emotions, i.e. fear of death.

- **Intellectual**: Yes, he is healthy as he has the capacity to think clearly and coherently. He can make decisions about his personal affairs and he can do his work.

- **Sexual**: Yes, he has an intimate and loving relationship with his partner.

- **Social**: Yes, he is healthy as he has a strong friendship circle.

- **Spiritual**: Yes, he reads the *Bible*, he has a religious faith and considers himself spiritually healthy, a view shared by his family and colleagues.

Overall, then, although his health professionals and his work colleagues may say he is not, Peter considers himself to be healthy.

Activity 1.2: Critical thinking (page 12)

All of them are health promotion activities. Consider the range of people involved and types of activity – education, prevention measures and policies. All will educate for health, prevent disease or protect the public.

Activity 1.3: Reflection (page 26)

The following theories and models may inform the programme's interventions:

- use epidemiology and demography to assess obesity as a health problem;

- assess the concepts of health of the client group;

- consider the social and cultural/educational background of your client group;

- what are the environmental issues/factors?

- examine local and national health policies;

- consider the infrastructure of health service provision;

- include interventions that address the needs of the young people;

- focus on equity;

- use Tannahill's model as a framework for planning, implementing and evaluating interventions;

- use Prochaska and DiClemente to ascertain the clients' stage of commitment and to assess progress.

Further reading

Naidoo, J and Wills, J (2010) *Developing Practice for Public Health and Health Promotion* (3rd edn). Oxford: Elsevier.

This is a good overview of health promotion, which also explains a range of health promotion models.

Ogden, J (2012) *Health Psychology: A Textbook* (5th edn). Milton Keynes: Open University Press.

This is a good review of health psychology theory and research.

Useful websites

www.who.int/publications/en/

This is a good website for keeping abreast of global health promotion developments.

https://www.gov.uk/government/latest?departments%5B%5D=department-of-health

Here you can get updates regarding the latest developments on a variety of health-related issues.

Chapter 2
Tackling lifestyle change

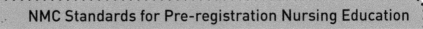
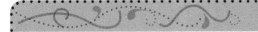

continued . . .

By entry to the register:

18. Discusses sensitive issues in relation to public health and provides appropriate advice and guidance to individuals, communities and populations, for example, contraception, substance misuse, smoking, obesity.

Cluster: Nutrition and fluid management

27. People can trust the newly registered graduate nurse to assist them to choose a diet that provides an adequate nutritional and fluid intake.

By entry to the register:

6. Uses knowledge of dietary, physical, social and psychological factors to inform practice, being aware of those that can contribute to poor diet, cause or be caused by ill health.

7. Supports people to make appropriate choices and changes to eating patterns, taking account of dietary preferences, religious and cultural requirements, treatment requirements and special diets needed for health reasons.

9. Discusses in a non-judgemental way how diet can improve health and the risks associated with not eating appropriately.

Chapter aims

By the end of this chapter you will be able to:

- locate and understand the current advice for healthy **lifestyle** choices;
- realise the social, psychological and political dimensions of targeting lifestyle for health improvement;
- begin working with patients on making healthy lifestyle choices.

Introduction

There is a confusion of information around healthy lifestyle choices. Some are well evidenced and clear and others seem to be difficult because the messages keep altering. As a nurse you need to have an overall understanding in order not only to guide patients when their lifestyles are causing ill health, but also to answer questions from patients and the public about healthy lifestyles generally. The NMC requires that all nurses support their patients' decision making and healthy lifestyle choices. You need to keep up to date with research evidence as it is presented through professional guidelines and campaign messages to the public. Obviously, as a professional, you need to understand the evidence behind these guidelines and messages in order to become a better practitioner with more credibility with patients and the public.

Case study: Choosing a healthy lifestyle is not easy

A district nurse was visiting an elderly patient with diabetes at her home when the husband of the patient suddenly said he had started eating olive oil spread because of the reports of it possibly lowering cholesterol levels in the blood. His wife joined in with the comment that he should be eating another particular spread (containing plant sterols) as this is advertised as definitely lowering cholesterol levels. She went on to suggest, however, that all fat is bad and he should be using only a scraping of any spread on his bread.

How did the district nurse tackle this?

- *First, she asked the husband to check the percentage of olive oil in the spread he was using. This was only 10 per cent, so he conceded that this was probably not worth it.*

- *Second, the nurse explained that the plant sterol and plant stanol spreads have been well researched and proven to lower blood cholesterol.*

- *But, third, she informed the couple that these need to be eaten in certain doses to be effective – a scraping would not be enough.*

It is not easy to make decisions about healthy lifestyles when the information is so complicated. Would you be able to help as the district nurse did?

This chapter offers a structure for you to think about tackling lifestyle change with patients. Any healthy lifestyle topic, whether multiple (such as healthy eating) or simple (such as salt in the diet), can be approached in this way. You can apply the structural approach to your favourite topics, and use it when a new topic is needed for your practice area. Figure 2.1 shows the areas you need to think about for each healthy lifestyle topic.

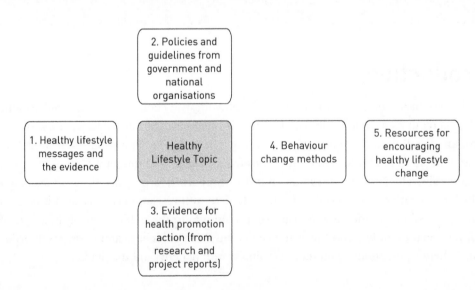

Figure 2.1: Areas to think about with healthy lifestyle topics

You need first to focus on and narrow down a healthy lifestyle topic. 'Sexual health' as a topic is too broad, and as a key word or phrase will give you too much information. Using more precise terminology such as 'safer sex' will narrow your search down, but 'condom use' will clearly focus more usefully. Similarly, you can narrow 'obesity' down to 'exercise' or 'losing weight' and 'healthy eating' down to 'fruit and vegetables'. Try to find a single, clear behaviour change to work on with patients as, in reality, people manage change more effectively in small steps. Once you have identified a topic, this chapter will guide you through each of the sections in boxes 1 to 5 of Figure 2.1 and explore the issues in each.

Before that, however, you need to be aware of the wider political decision making concerned with healthy lifestyle choices.

The politics of healthy lifestyle choices

In modern health promotion terms there is always a tension between people making healthy choices and government providing the essential opportunities and structures for people to have choices. The WHO recognised the need to shift the emphasis away from always assuming it is the individual's responsibility towards sharing the responsibility with government-organised provision. (See Chapter 1, page 14, for details of the Ottawa Charter, which recognised the responsibility of governments to make living environments that support individual and community skills in making decisions and choices for health.) At the time in the 1980s the UK, under right-wing Conservative government rule, did not acknowledge that the state shared responsibility and tended to place responsibility on individuals for their health choices, their own health, and therefore ill health. The election of a left-wing Labour government in 1997 resulted in a health policy of shared responsibility and a focus on partnership between people, organisations and government. The government health policy in 2004 (also Labour) changed to a shift in emphasis further towards the idea of empowering people's choices by providing supportive environments. One of the clearest examples is the ban on smoking in enclosed public places, where the intent was not only to protect the public from the effects of passive smoking, but also to provide better social and environmental opportunities for smokers to quit and non-smokers not to start. The public health white paper, *Choosing Health* (DH, 2004b), intended to refocus from major disease targets to lifestyle issues and to promise more central government intervention to support healthy lifestyle choices. The targets named in this white paper were: reducing the numbers of people who smoke, reducing obesity and improving diet and nutrition, increasing exercise, encouraging and supporting sensible drinking, improving sexual health and improving mental health.

In 2010 the coalition government of the Conservative and Liberal Democrat parties, right wing and centre, produced their own white paper for England, which replaced the previous one. *Healthy Lives, Healthy People* (DH, 2010b) declared that centralisation had failed and promised a radical new approach, focusing on work in local communities, led by local government (which they called 'localisation'). The government intended to tackle the promotion of healthy lifestyles through recognising the difficulties and inequalities people face, and by providing educational, social and financial support for people's healthy choices. The targets of their white paper were given not as topics but as intentions to work in ways that address root causes of ill health. Wales, Scotland and Northern Ireland have their own strategies, generally following the national trends in health needs.

Healthy lifestyle messages and the evidence

Going now to the sections of Figure 2.1, remember your chosen lifestyle topic and apply the following ideas for finding the evidence.

Interpreting the message

We tend to be bombarded from all directions by messages that tell us to do this and that, or not to do something. Have you ever tried to collect them all and put them together as a set of ideas for working with patients, or even your own family?

Here are some of the messages you may have come across:

- eat five portions of fruit and vegetables a day;
- take enough exercise;
- eat less sugar;
- practise safer sex;
- eat less fat overall, but particularly saturated fat;
- don't smoke at all;
- have a social life;
- wear safety equipment;
- drink a sensible level of alcohol.

But do you know the detailed instructions related to the messages, and do you know the evidence behind them?

Start with the message to eat five portions of fruit and vegetables a day. When the 5-a-day campaign was launched in 2003 with this simple message, people were confused about portions and what exactly counted as fruit and vegetables. The campaign was adapted to try to get a more detailed message across but, overall, this has not been as successful as was hoped. It may have been due to a kind of campaign fatigue and needed refreshing completely. In 2009, Change4Life (www.nhs.uk/change4life) was launched with the slogan 'Eat Well, Move More, Live Longer'. This **social marketing** approach to tackle obesity and general health aims to give people more help with acting on the messages. The campaign is expanding and is based currently on healthy behaviour messages, colourfully presented in a simple format aimed at families. The campaign uses magazine and TV adverts, social media and partnership with, for example, the British Heart Foundation and Kelloggs. There is a local supporters' network for schools, hospitals and health professionals you can join, and resources are available. In 2016 Public Health England launched 'One You', a campaign aimed at middle-aged adults (40 to 60) for the first time, targeting this group in a similar way to Change4Life by encouraging people to eat well, drink less, exercise more and give up smoking. When people enter www.nhs.uk/oneyou they are asked to complete a quiz that personalises the information on healthy lifestyle. Public Health England suggest that 40 per cent of all deaths in this age group in England are related to behavioural choices. The campaign has been criticised as patronising. Have a look and see what you think of this new resource.

Another message that causes controversy is the one about sensible drinking (alcohol). Some adults will remember that the safe number of units of alcohol suggested for men and women daily has changed over the years. They will tell you that 'the government can't make up its mind, so what does it matter?' New guidelines for alcohol consumption were introduced in 2016. There is no longer a differentiation between risks and limits for men and women. The guide for both is 14 units a week over three days. One alcohol unit is measured as 10ml or 8g of pure alcohol. This equals one 25ml single measure of whisky (ABV 40 per cent), or a third of a pint of beer (ABV 5–6 per cent) or half a standard (175ml) glass of red wine (ABV 12 per cent). It is also stated that there is no safe level of consumption. The risk of cancers in particular is emphasised and confirmed by the World Cancer Research Fund. See the Drinkaware website for recent changes. Drinking a lot of alcohol at once (binge drinking) is dangerous. It can lead to liver and brain damage, cause accidents and encourage violent crime. Binge drinking is considered to be drinking six units for women and eight units for men, at any one time. (Further information can be found on the website www.drinkaware.co.uk)

Another strong piece of advice released in 2016 was the message to avoid vitamin D deficiency through nutrition, sunlight and supplementation. We are now advised to obtain at least 10 micrograms of vitamin D a day. Supplementation is advised, at least in autumn and winter, and all year for those people with darker skin and/or those who do not have much exposure to sunlight (www.gov.government/publications/sacn-vitamin-d-and-health-report).

Finally in this section, there was a change to the educational device of a picture of a plate to show healthy eating. You may have been using this already. The educational device of a plate was first launched in 1994 as The Balance of Good Health. This was amended, after more research, and became the Eatwell Plate in 2007. These two 'plates' were replaced in 2016 by the Eatwell Guide (another plate, but not called that). Criticisms of this device continue; its lack of strong evidence and cultural awareness for example. The main recent changes include new ideas about sugars, carbohydrates and fats. The current diagram shows increased fruit and vegetables, no fruit juice, added water and emphasises unsaturated fats, as well as providing information about food labelling and calories. There is an interactive version showing these changes on www.nhs.uk/Livewell/Goodfood/Pages/the-eatwell-guide.aspx

---

Activity 2.1   *Research and finding evidence*

Now think of a healthy lifestyle topic and do the same investigation of the message. For example, how much and what sort of exercise should a well adult be doing and why?

- What is the message – exactly?
- What details would someone ask about the message? How does someone follow it?
- What is the evidence? Why are people being asked to do this? What does this choice prevent, and how?

An outline answer is provided at the end of the chapter.

Finding the latest and most evidence-based message for a healthy lifestyle topic is an important part of the nurse's role in health promotion. In addition, adaptations to the message will be needed.

Adapting the message

The messages need to be adapted for everyone depending on people's wide variety of circumstances. Most campaigns are aware of this and you will find variations for children, the differently able, the elderly, etc. Perhaps not in the campaign information, but in the evidence from projects professionals have published, will be variations you can apply to different groups, such as those with ethnic differences, religious constraints and social disadvantages. What is not explored so well is the variation you may need for patients with existing illnesses (both physical and mental).

Activity 2.2   *Critical thinking*

Draw up a list of possible variations your patient has that would mean you have to modify a message, such as to eat less fat.

- age – children and older adults have different needs;
- gender – women and men may have specific issues to do with physiology or social norms;
- religion – several religions have constraints on individual choices;
- culture – people across the world have different ways of living;
- income level – this will link to social circumstance, housing and access to a healthy lifestyle;
- education level – not something we tend to measure, but think about the patient's ability to learn;
- effects of illness – the patient's illness, or psychological responses to it, will affect learning and the ability to change lifestyle.

Modify the message to suit.

An outline answer is provided at the end of the chapter.

In addition to understanding the evidence supporting the healthy lifestyle messages, you need to consider the origins of the messages and the related guidance for their use. The next section goes on to discuss this.

Policies and guidelines from government and national organisations

This is the next section of Figure 2.1 to be considered. The UK government, its departments, agencies and partners produce policies and guidelines on all health issues. The healthy lifestyle topics sometimes appear alone (smoking) or in groups (drugs, alcohol and smoking) or are integrated into disease-related strategies (coronary heart disease and cancers). The policies come in different guises. There are laws (smoking ban in public), white papers (various aspects of public health), national service frameworks (for example, diabetes) and strategic plans (for example, sexual health). These are usually applicable across the UK but you need to be aware of countrywide variations.

When you are looking into a healthy lifestyle topic, the Department of Health is a good place to start as it originates or commissions so many of these documents (use the website www.gov.uk/government/organisations/department-of-health). Charity organisations also produce guidelines and are reliable (for example, Diabetes UK, British Heart Foundation); some are official partners of the government and take the lead (such as Drinkaware, the Terrence Higgins Trust, Breast Cancer Care). You could also just use an internet search engine to find documents on your topic – in which case you must be careful to look at the organisation name on the url and only rely on government or other official sites such as charities and professional organisations. Don't, for example, make the mistake of using a commercial company site for guidance when they are in the business of selling products. Websites set up as personal opinion and radical anti-establishment outlets can be used to make you think, but do be professional about how you use the information. Tell patients the same thing, and only use reliable references in your academic work.

Table 2.1 shows some of the current national documents that guide practice in healthy lifestyle promotion. It does not include the very useful NHS documents that focus on care provision but that also address some prevention issues (such as the national service frameworks). Remember to look for updates, evaluations and reviews of any strategy you are researching.

What you must do is find the follow-up to the document you are researching. There may be a further document with more details of action to be taken, or an evaluation of the strategy some time after its launch. Also, when governments change after elections expect new strategic plans to be drawn up. When you go into the Department of Health website, the latest news will be there and you can see that some of the most popular documents are posted on the front page. Use the website's search box to find any document you are looking for.

Having looked at the national strategies and guidelines for healthy lifestyle topics, you may have found some helpful ideas for practice in the examples given by the documents. Next you need to move on to the effectiveness of health promotion practice itself. The next step in the structure in Figure 2.1 is to show that your methods of practice are evidence-based.

Activity 2.3   *Research and finding evidence*

Go to the Department of Health website (www.gov.uk/government/organisations/department-of-health). Click on public health (www.gov.uk/government/topics/public-health) and you will find a page that shows the latest news. You can search for other topics and publications from here. Search for a health topic that interests you such as, for example, Physical Activity, and follow through to the documents available.

Some of the documents listed will inevitably be either old ones or merely press releases and letters from the Department. However, this is a useful way to find out what is published and the website puts them in order of usefulness.

As this activity relies on your own research, there is no outline answer at the end of the chapter.

Table 2.1 National (led by England) guidelines for some healthy lifestyle topics

Lifestyle topic	Date	Guideline	Organisation
General – current public health white paper	2010	*Healthy Lives, Healthy People: Our strategy for public health in England.*	Department of Health
General – children	2007	*Healthy Lives, Brighter Futures: The strategy for children and young people's health.*	Department of Health
Obesity	2011 (updated 2015)	*Healthy Lives, Healthy People: A call to action on obesity in England.*	Department of Health
Healthy eating	2009	Change4Life	Department of Health
Sexual health	2013	*A Framework for Sexual Health Improvement in England.*	Department of Health
	2010	*Teenage Pregnancy Strategy: Beyond 2010.*	Teenage Pregnancy Unit, Department for Education
Drugs	2010 (reviewed 2014-15)	*Reducing Demand, Restricting Supply, Building Recovery: Supporting people to live a drug-free life.*	HM Government
Smoking	2011	*Healthy Lives, Healthy People: A tobacco control plan for England.*	Department of Health
Mental health	2011	*No Health Without Mental Health: A cross-governmental health outcomes strategy for people of all ages.*	Department of Health
Physical activity	2004	*At Least Five a Week: Evidence from the Chief Medical Officer.*	Department of Health
	2009	*Be Active, Be Healthy.*	Department of Health
Alcohol	2012	*The Government's Alcohol Strategy.*	Home Office

Evidence for health promotion action

You need to find out if the health messages and the national guidelines are working. This section looks at the effectiveness of health promotion, which delivers the message to improve healthy lifestyles.

Health promotion can be structured as a combination of health education, prevention services (primary, secondary and tertiary) and policies to protect health (Tannahill, 2009). These three aspects should be based on the best available evidence from research, from national campaigns and from evaluation of local practice.

Concept summary: Tannahill's model of health promotion

This model explains Tannahill's (1985 and 2009) view that health promotion is a mixture of the following three areas of activity.

- **Health education** – teaching people about health and how to live healthily. This is done largely through schools and the media, although as health professionals you will also have a role in this.
- **Prevention** – providing services to prevent disease, such as immunisation, screening and support to live well with an existing disease.
- **Health protection** – which Tannahill sees as setting laws, policies and allocating money to promote health.

The three areas overlap with each other so that health education can help prevent disease, and health protection can agree policy for education and prevention services. The model is useful for making you think of all possible aspects of a topic – such as smoking:

- health education in schools and by the NHS at www.smokefree.nhs.uk;
- prevention through smoking cessation classes and nicotine replacement;
- health protection from the ban on smoking in enclosed public places and restrictions on advertising and sales.

The model shows the interrelationships between teaching people about healthy lifestyles (health education), understanding what is being prevented and how (prevention) and the policy environment in which choices are made (health protection). Tannahill's model enables health professionals to think of a whole approach to health promotion for groups of people with similar needs. Now apply Tannahill's model to your work with people on healthy lifestyles.

Activity 2.4 **Critical thinking**

Think of how health promotion can be constructed for a healthy lifestyle topic such as, for example, oral health.

- Health education – What would you teach patients?
- Prevention services – What would you advise patients to do about preventing disease? Who could help them?
- What can you find out about protective policies and national guidelines?

An outline answer is provided at the end of the chapter.

The model, as you can see, attempts to cover the potential whole range of initiatives to improve health: educating people, providing prevention services and setting policies to protect health. It should enable you to plan interventions across that range within your practice.

Many health promotion initiatives are also structured around these three aspects, even though they may not say so. Local initiatives (often called projects) are set up on one or more topics, for example tackling obesity in children, foot health for the elderly, healthy eating for long-term mentally ill people or a youth-focused project tackling a mixture of issues, such as alcohol, drugs, sex and safety in the street. This kind of work gives evidence that is not from scientific research, but is seen as collecting evidence from interventions and is usually evaluated with collections of data that are a mixture of quantitative and qualitative responses.

Evidence for health promotion is often not strong. Research using randomised controlled trials (the best sort of evidence) is rarely conducted in the case of setting up an initiative involving, for example, sex education classes or after-school sports or campaigns on using less salt. They are difficult because different groups have to be organised so that a strict comparison can be made when the only difference between them is the intervention itself. Imagine having two groups of children in a school where one group has swimming classes and one does not. The children in the non-swimming group may go swimming with their families, so the difference is lost. Also, it would be seen as unfair and ethically unjustifiable to deprive one group of an intervention when it is known to be beneficial. Imagine a group of obese children in one community where half of them join a special exercise class and the other half get no extra help.

Clearly there are some instances where strictly scientific research methods could work: nicotine replacement therapy, cancer screening or weight-loss programmes for adults. The ethical issues remain but at least the intervention itself can be controlled. Some research compares two or more interventions such as different diets. The National Institute for Health and Care Excellence (NICE) publishes the best evidence for a range of public health topics (as well as the better known work they do on drug treatments). To find these documents go to the NICE website, www. nice.org.uk, and look for your topic or look at the public health guidance available. There is a general document on behaviour change (NICE, 2007) and guidance on topics such as alcohol, obesity, physical activity, sexual health and smoking.

Evidence from projects in health promotion is often hard to find. Some edited textbooks will have chapters written by people who report on their project; some journals will have similar articles. In England local authorities (since April 2013), and elsewhere in the UK local community health organisations working with their local authority, generate and operate local initiatives to improve health. Finally, a scholarly approach should lead you into doing a literature search using search engines and journal databases. What you will find is a good and wide professional literature on health promotion research and health promotion intervention projects/initiatives. You will need to refine your keywords to narrow your search to the most relevant articles.

Having by this time found out the details of the health messages, looked at the national guidelines around them and read some evidence from projects in the literature, you are now ready to plan interventions for patients. The next section examines ways to change behaviour.

Behaviour change methods

All health promotion can be seen as having the aim of promoting **health behaviour** change. Even when using Tannahill's model, it is about:

- education to promote behaviour change;
- promoting a change to preventive behaviour and using preventive services;
- being aware of the effect of social and environmental constraints on change and also the promotion of healthy choices through healthy policy setting.

Behaviour change models

No one makes choices or changes behaviour in isolation. There are internal factors such as a person's upbringing, or influences on beliefs and attitudes from general education, culture and family. There are external factors such as environment, social contacts, religion and income. How people make health behaviour changes has been the subject of much theory and research. There are models of behaviour change based on beliefs and knowledge (cognition models), social influence (social cognition models) and empowerment (empowerment models), all of which are helpful for you to consider in order to help patients change their behaviour.

Cognition models focus on the thinking of the individual, so beliefs, attitudes and values are most influential in his or her decision making. This will mean that, as a nurse, you work with those beliefs or work to change them, either to help a patient to develop a way of adapting the health message (losing weight on a personal choice of preferred food) or to convince the patient to alter his or her beliefs (to try a different way of eating from that 'set' by family or perhaps by bad experiences). The limitations to these models are that merely tailoring the behaviour change advice to beliefs only makes people 'think' of suitable changes (hence the cognition). They do not enable or empower people to change. This is referred to as the gap between 'intention to change behaviour' and 'changing behaviour'.

Social cognition models introduce the influence of other people on a patient's behaviour, so that the patient may worry about not being 'normal' or being seen to be 'fussy' or 'picky' if she or he chooses things that friends would not. Men giving up drinking alcohol may be ridiculed by their mates for choosing 'girly' soft drinks. Sometimes the fear factor is strong, either stopping healthy behaviour (fear of looking fat in an exercise class) or promoting the behaviour (reading about famous young women dying of cervical cancer may encourage attendance for smear tests). The limitations to these models are that, despite showing what other people do and think of certain behaviours, they still do not enable people to be empowered to change. The gap between intention and behaviour is not closed.

Empowerment models (see also Chapter 5) make the assumption that the previous two types of behaviour change theory do not take into account how hard it is for people to make decisions to change. Empowerment models show how people need to become empowered through their own previous actions (they learn how to be successful) or need to be empowered by others – in this case by you as a nurse. The NMC standards include the role of the nurse in empowering patients in their decision making. Empowerment does not come because more knowledge is gained, so giving your patient all the information will only go so far. Empowerment is also about being able to weigh up or judge the information – empowering the patient to decide for themselves, even when new or conflicting information is released. Further, empowerment is boosting the patient's own belief in her or his abilities to make decisions. You know yourself how difficult this is when other people do not believe that you can do it. Not least, empowerment is about 'making space' for the patient, ensuring that his or her voice is heard and opinions valued. Some would call this a true partnership with the patient, enabling the person to move on from thinking and knowing what other people think, to that risky step of making a decision to change. This may go some way to closing the intention–behaviour gap. However, an empowered person may still have difficulty, even having made the decision, in actually making the change.

A model of behaviour change that purports to cross over and include all the theories above is the *transtheoretical stages of change model* (Prochaska and DiClemente, 1982); see Table 2.2. The idea is that people go through stages and the health professional can enable progress through these stages. It is important to realise that this alters the way a nurse can enable behaviour change. It is foolish to simplistically imagine that the patient will start to change as soon as he or she has had a teaching session on the ward or in the practice, and then take on board the goal of change such as giving up smoking. The authors of the model suggest that the goal of a health professional, given his or her limited time with each patient, need only be to move the patient from one stage to the next, since expecting to complete the cycle any time soon is unrealistic.

The model describes how people go through stages where at first they do not consider changing their health behaviour (pre-contemplation), then start to think they should (contemplation).

The next stage is to get ready to change by reading and investigating how to change (preparation), followed by taking the first step in trying a new behaviour (making a change). At several stages, people may relapse and go back to old behaviours, commonly when they have tried something and it has not worked for them. Eventually, though, the model describes how people maintain a new healthy behaviour and stay changed. Each stage is not easy to reach from the previous one and how you as a nurse can help is in finding ways to motivate someone to take another step along the model or go back into the process from a relapse.

Table 2.2 Prochaska and DiClemente's transtheoretical stages of change model (adapted from Prochaska and DiClemente, 1982)

Stage of change	What happens	Moving someone to the next stage
Pre-contemplation	The patient is unaware that a change is needed and/or has no intention of changing in the future.	Something to attract and alert the patient is required – perhaps a fun event with a free gift or a graphic, fear-inducing warning.
Contemplation	Some realisation is occurring and the patient expresses that 'I really ought to do this – some time.'	The patient needs to be helped to make a plan. The idea that there are many ways of changing can be introduced. Sometimes the story of a successful role model can help: 'If he can do it, so can I.'
Preparing to change	Now the patient is seeking information about changing, asking questions, reading about it – not changing yet though, but still looking for support and reassurance.	Without causing information overload, ideas are required. Provide a range of options and a range of sources of information – leaflets, websites, free introductory sessions. Encourage the choice of something to try out. Negotiate a start date or the investigation will take a long time.
Making a change	The decision is made to try a new way to make a change. It may be quite tentative and dependent on the weather or who goes to the group. The change is tried out; for a while it will be seen as a test period.	Now is the time for praise and building self-esteem. Listen to the patient as she or he describes her or his experience of change. Congratulate the patient and encourage her or him to keep it up. At the same time you can reassure the patient that one slip-up does not mean failure.

(Continued)

Table 2.2 (*Continued*)

Stage of change	What happens	Moving someone to the next stage
Relapse	This does not always happen. The patient does not like what he or she is trying out – 'It doesn't work', 'I don't like it', 'They were not nice to me.'	This is the potential failure. Work with the patient on what to do next. It may be that he or she needs to try an entirely new method as this one did not suit. It may be that the patient only needs to be told again that one day of bad behaviour does not mean that he or she cannot start again.
Staying changed	The particular new health behaviour has been established. The patient is convinced it is working, in fact becomes rather proud and tells everybody.	The job is not finished yet. The patient now needs to complete his or her empowerment. The patient is successful and needs praise, and also needs to use his or her new power. Try asking the person to speak to other patients about his or her success. Ask the person for suggestions for helping other patients.
	On to the next change? This model is an upward-climbing spiral.	The successful, empowered patient tries a change in another aspect of her or his health.

Because of the great difficulty people have making changes, this model is still criticised for not doing enough to close the intention–behaviour gap that exists between the stages of 'preparation' and 'making a change'. Some professionals consider the way to close the gap is through helping the person to action plan for change.

Activity 2.5   *Communication*

Consider a patient from the following list:

- a 50-year-old woman with diabetes;
- a 30-year-old man with a personality disorder;
- a 14-year-old girl with asthma;
- a 24-year-old man who has a learning disability.

How would you work with them on their smoking cessation at each stage of the Prochaska and DiClemente model?

An outline answer is provided at the end of the chapter.

Understanding and using these behaviour change models may help you to understand how theory can work in practice. Seeing how people progress from one stage of the stages of change model to another will enable you to set realistic goals in health promotion, rather than expecting immediate new health behaviour.

Behaviour change techniques

In addition to the behaviour change models above, there are other techniques that you might want to consider using. These have been developed mainly within the medical profession as tools for use by general practitioners and, of course, other health professionals have adopted their use.

Motivational interviewing (Rollnick et al., 2008) is an interpersonal style rather than a structured model. It has four general principles:

- express empathy with the problem and the need to change;
- develop discrepancy (make people understand the differences and the advantages and disadvantages) between current behaviour and desired change;
- accept resistance to change as normal;
- support self-efficacy and autonomy in changing behaviour.

In this way motivational interviewers can show the patient that her or his problem is understandable, that the need to change is evident, that reluctance to change is natural and that the patient can do it. Motivational interviewing tends to stand alone as a technique and is used very often by medical professionals. The goal is often to empower, and as a nurse you can adopt the technique as a means to show the patient the same things.

Brief intervention (Babor and Higgins-Biddle, 2001) is a term used to indicate the time available and taken, rather than any particular technique. It can also be referred to as solution-focused brief therapy and is intended to keep the session directly on the issue of the behaviour change needed. Most of the writers in this field suggest that it has the following principles:

- to raise awareness of the risks in current behaviour;
- to emphasise the patient's responsibility in making a change;
- to give advice to change;
- to make suggestions for strategies for change;
- to encourage goal setting and action planning for change.

Brief intervention can be the focus used in any of the previous theories and models, as a means to take the patient quite quickly to a decision point and action. It is used very often in alcohol behaviour and emotional issues. It is slightly more direct than motivational interviewing and tends to challenge the patient to action. The goal is to make change happen soon as the risks are high.

A totally different approach to health behaviour change has been recently reintroduced to the debate. *Financial incentives* to change behaviour have been proposed, particularly in the areas of obesity and weight loss. In a scheme backed by the NHS called Weight Wins, run by a private company, people are offered cash for losing pounds and for keeping them off. There have been suggestions for using incentives for other topics, such as compliance with drug treatments, contraception uptake, screening attendance and smoking cessation. The incentives need not be cash, but could be vouchers for food or donations to charities. Incentives used in smoking cessation have so far shown no increase in successful quitting, but there has been an increase in numbers of people joining smoking cessation groups.

NICE is unsure about the effectiveness of incentives and has set up a consultation around the issue. It feels that their use could be divisive, rewarding people for what should be done anyway and unfair to people who do it by themselves. People who argue for the use of incentives feel that any method of improving health is worthwhile. NICE has recommended further research into incentives.

Resources for encouraging healthy lifestyle

The final step in Figure 2.1 is for you to think of resources in your chosen topic. Now you have a better idea of the messages you want to deliver, the policy background, evidence for health promotion and ways to address behaviour change, you need to consider what resources to use with patients. You can, to an extent, rely on your own knowledge and skills to explain, to write instructions, to draw diagrams and so on. However, there are many sources of useful teaching materials to help you and to provide for patients and clients to use for themselves.

First, think of what sort of resource material would be useful to your patient group and care environment.

- Leaflets are reading material and not everyone reads, or they may learn better through other means.

- Posters can have impact and may attract the attention of people at the pre-contemplation stage. They can make an interesting and eye-catching display.

- Websites that the patients can access are becoming more useful. Children are particularly computer aware and 'silver surfers' are on the increase.

- Films on DVD are ideal for a group session or for continual showing in a waiting area.

- Models of parts of the body, food portion sizes, lungs damaged by smoking, etc. can make things clearer than a diagram. Equipment such as tape measures indicating healthy waist size, pedometers and condom demonstrator models can all be found.

- Increasingly, mobile phone 'apps' are being used, which are mainly produced by some commercial companies working with slimming for example, and there is a British Heart Foundation recipe finder available free from iTunes. The NHS is developing a library of safe and trusted health apps, including support for management of conditions and healthy lifestyle choices (www.nhs.uk/tools/pages/toolslibrary.aspx).

- Finally, when you are teaching a group about a healthy lifestyle, try to make it fun and give free gifts such as apples, toothbrushes and smiley face badges.

Remember that all teaching resource materials are more effective when accompanied by health professional input. Work with the patient to personalise the resource. See Chapter 4 for more information and advice on teaching patients.

You need to understand where to get resources from. Again, as at the beginning of the chapter, think of a health message and locate organisations that produce related resources.

Activity 2.6   *Research and finding evidence*

Using a message about being aware of stress, contact your local community health organisation, or local authority (in England), which has the remit to support you in your area of practice.

- Is there a government official organisation for this topic?
- Is there a day or week or month for the topic across the country or the world?
- Is there a charity organisation involved (it may not be exactly on the healthy lifestyle topic, but on a related preventable disease)?
- Is there a commercial organisation that you can officially ask for help? Be careful here because you do not want to advertise and you must not go outside your employer's purchasing contracts.
- What other resources can you get free? What is the cost involved if not?

An outline answer is provided at the end of the chapter.

There are many possible resources for health promotion, but you will have to work at obtaining them, as they are not located conveniently. Further guidance on managing resources in practice is given in Chapter 7.

Having looked at all the sections on the original structure in Figure 2.1, you should have a good idea of how to put together information and methods for healthy lifestyle topics. Consider the topic you chose at the beginning of the chapter: think of the evidence for the message, the policies involved, the evidence for health promotion being done, the behaviour change methods you can use and finally the resources available. One area left to explore is that of the nurse's own healthy lifestyle choices.

Nurses as healthy role models

The Prime Minister's Commission on the Future of Nursing and Midwifery in England (2010) reported that nurses should be role models for healthy living, and take responsibility for their own health. The International Council of Nurses made a similar statement on International Nurses Day in 2010.

There were various responses to the statements, mostly agreeing with the need to be healthy, but refuting the idea of role modelling as it may be seen as pretending to be better than the patient. Imagine what the patient may feel being helped by a nurse who shows extremely healthy behaviour – admiration or inferiority, aspiration or defeat? It is interesting that this imperative to become a role model is often directed at health professionals, whereas it would be unusual to expect a teacher never to have failed an exam or a counsellor never to have had an emotional problem. Perhaps we should recognise that nurses are as imperfect as anyone else and that what they can role model is not perfect behaviour but the ability to find things out, to be doing something about a problem and to be aware of the risks.

Take smoking, for example: if you are a smoker the patient can either relate to you or say that you can't help. If you are a non-smoker the patient can either emulate you or say you don't know what it's like. If you are a smoker who has quit, the patient may either admire you or say it was easier for you for some reason. The point is that you can and should be able to help a smoker to begin to quit whatever your personal behaviour. What you can model is having the facts, understanding the risks and knowing where to get help.

Chapter summary

This chapter has explored the issues involved in nurses working to promote health through tackling change towards healthy lifestyles. There are several themes under discussion, including the political dimension to healthy lifestyles and the difficulty of finding the evidence and the support needed for people to change behaviour. The role of nurses has been coordinated into a structure that is designed to help you gather the information you need to work with healthy lifestyle topics. This structure includes the understanding of healthy lifestyle messages, national policies, evidence for effective health promotion, health behaviour change and resources to help you help your patients.

Activities: brief outline answers

Activity 2.1: Research and finding evidence (page 33)

The exercise message is 'at least five a week'.

- At least 30 minutes a day of at least moderate-intensity physical activity on five or more days of the week. This can be one session or several short sessions of at least 10 minutes, or structured sessions of sports, for example. All exercise helps with weight management. For bone health, activities that produce high physical stresses on the bones are necessary. Exercise will also help to protect against cardiovascular disease, cancer, type 2 diabetes and obesity.

- Older adults should take particular care to keep moving through daily activity and do specific activities to improve strength, coordination and balance.

- Children and young people should achieve a total of at least 60 minutes of at least moderate-intensity physical activity each day. At least twice a week this should include activities to improve bone health (activities that produce high physical stresses on the bones), muscle strength and flexibility. This helps to prevent risk factors for disease, avoidance of weight gain, achieving a high-peak bone mass and mental well-being.

Activity 2.2: Critical thinking (page 34)

The message is to eat less fat, especially saturated fat – no more than 30g a day for men and 20g a day for women.

- Children should have less saturated fat than adults. However, a low-fat diet isn't suitable for children under five as they need the nutrients. Older people who are frail or underweight should not have a low-fat diet either.

- Some methods of cooking are traditionally high fat using, for example, ghee (clarified butter) or palm oil, both of which are saturated fats.

- When a family has a low income they tend to choose the cheaper supermarket food and the easy ready-made food. This limited set of choices is usually high in fat.

- Have you tried to work out from the labels how much fat is in your food? Labels give either a gram weight of fat or a percentage. However, you also have to work out the total fat and the saturated fat. This requires a level of reading and mathematical ability.

- People trying to lower their blood cholesterol are advised to lower total fats and saturated fats in their diets. There is currently much controversy as to whether a weight-reducing diet should be low fat or low carbohydrate. A very low-fat diet can lead to poor levels of hormones and affect fertility and brain function.

Activity 2.4: Critical thinking (page 38)

Health education:

- teaching knowledge of teeth and gum health and disease – fluoride, acid foods;
- demonstrating the practice of flossing, brushing and tongue cleaning;
- enabling behaviour change by motivating and empowering.

Preventive services:

- fluoride added to tap water;
- regular visits to a dentist;
- self-screening bleeding gums, pain and signs of cavities.

Protective guidelines.

- Do you know if your local water is fluoridised?

- Should you use fluoride toothpaste? Should a child?

- The British Dental Association now recommends using straws with fizzy drinks, not rinsing after using fluoride toothpaste, and ending a meal with alkaline food such as cheese, not fruit.

Activity 2.5: Communication (page 43)

There will probably be more similarities than differences between these people. Each of them may have fears, a lack of awareness and a varying level of ability to make a decision. The following shows some ideas for the more likely variations.

- Older people may resent being told what to do and may rely on traditional ways or think they know things because they are experienced. Having illnesses just means getting older and causes more resentment. Older people may feel it is 'too late to change'. They may not respond well to having to read more or expose their problems in a group. Try persuading older people to change because of the small differences it can make to their health such as, for example, being less breathless or having fewer chest infections in winter.

- People with mental illness often have no insight into the risks they are running. They can be inattentive and unresponsive to advice. Habitual behaviours such as smoking are frequently part of the whole make-up of the person and may be multiple (alcohol and drugs perhaps as well). They may have difficulty making decisions or have little insight into the risks. Try to help them to see relevant benefits to their lives such as, for example, having more money to spend on clothes or leisure items. Focus on healthy eating if they are interested in that, instead of smoking, reminding people that their appetites will improve if they quit smoking. In a way, this is similar to using incentives, which may also work.

- Teenagers tend to resent having to manage long-term illness. They also cannot see the point of health advice for what they see as 'old people's illnesses'. Smoking may be 'cool' in their group and the opinions of their peers are very influential. Some ways of quitting are more difficult than others; going to a group where there are only adults is not very encouraging. Try to find age-appropriate learning materials. Using rewards is popular in this age group, as is concentrating on appearance and attractiveness instead of long-term risks.

- For people with learning disabilities, the approach needs to be at the appropriate cognitive level such as, for example, using simple messages, demonstrations that are close to reality and clear associations of cigarettes with coughing. Metaphors and stylised material are not easily understood. Supervision and guidance are vital as attention may vary and repetition of your input will be needed.

When dealing with the stages, these differences can interfere with your work. Some patients will take much longer than others to go from stage to stage and the final goal of quitting smoking may not be attained.

Activity 2.6: Research and finding evidence (page 45)

- You may find that you can get an allocation of free government leaflets and posters from your local community health organisation or local authority. You can ask if any of the health promotion staff there can help you.

- The Department of Health provides leaflets and posters on a range of health topics. You need to go to the DH at www.orderline.dh.gov.uk and set up a customer number for yourself.

- World Mental Health Day is 10 October, National Stress Awareness Day is 6 November and Anger Awareness Week is in December. Use a search engine to look for health events specific to your work – you may find local events too. MIND (www.mind.org.uk) and the Royal College of Psychiatrists (www.rcpsych.ac.uk) are two organisations that produce resources. They may only be online or may cost money for bulk orders. If you are going to set up an information stall, or run a small campaign across a health facility, you could ask for other types of resources or for sponsorship to buy them. Your care organisation's catering company would be a good place to start. It may be persuaded to donate fruit (bananas for relaxation?) or to sponsor activities. There are stress balls for relaxation but they cost a lot of money. The local gym or complementary therapy practice may be persuaded to give trial sessions and advertise its facilities at the same time.

Further reading

Hutchfield, K (2010) *Information Skills for Nursing Students.* Exeter: Learning Matters.

This is a good instruction book for using information technology.

Ogden, J (2012) *Health Psychology: A Textbook* (5th edn). Milton Keynes: Open University Press.

This is a good basic review of a wide range of health behaviour change theories with critical comments about their effective applications.

Useful websites

www.bhf.org.uk

The British Heart Foundation website is very useful for information about healthy hearts (and long-term conditions). There are also plenty of resources for teaching schoolchildren about hearts and blood pressure, etc.

www.drinkaware.co.uk

This is the site for alcohol information and the national campaign led by a partnership of organisations, including the alcohol industry.

www.nhs.uk/change4life

This is the government's main campaign for healthy lifestyles, eating, exercise and alcohol.

www.nhs.uk

This is the public access page of the NHS 'choice agenda' created by the Labour government in 2008. This is the website to which people are directed in public libraries.

www.nhs.uk/smokefree

This is the main website to help people stop smoking.

www.nice.org.uk

This is the National Institute for Health and Care Excellence, where you can find (in the public health section) the best evidence for health promotion interventions as collated so far.

www.talktofrank.com

This is the current drugs awareness organisation, useful for information on all recreational drugs and resources for use in practice.

Chapter 3
Encouraging health screening

....
NMC Standards for Pre-registration Nursing Education

This chapter will address the following competencies:

Domain 3: Nursing practice and decision-making

5. All nurses must understand public health principles, priorities and practice in order to recognise and respond to the major causes and social determinants of health, illness and health inequalities. They must use a range of information and data to assess the needs of people, groups, communities and populations and work to improve health, well-being and experiences of healthcare; secure equal access to health screening, health promotion and health care; and promote social inclusion.
....

Chapter aims

By the end of this chapter you will be able to:

*   give an account of screening for ill health, as part of secondary prevention of ill health within health promotion;
*   understand the importance of health screening;
*   identify and list the range of screening types available in the UK;
*   recognise how nurses may be able to discuss health screening with patients.

Introduction

Screening is the process of undertaking particular tests on apparently healthy, symptom-free people, who may be at risk of a specific disease or condition of which they are unaware. This testing of people is carried out on a large scale and people are invited from particular age or gender groups.

As a nurse you need to have an understanding of how members of the population will be offered the chance to have health screening and what kinds of screening are available in the UK. You must be aware of how this could make a contribution to their health and well-being and you should be able to answer questions that some of your patients may have. Nurses must also be aware about some of the reasons patients may choose whether or not to accept the invitation for screening. The subject of screening is regularly discussed in the media, and some health issues can be given a high profile. Patients may turn to you to discuss the various topics, in which case you need to have a clear understanding of the guidelines behind the screening programmes. This chapter considers the role of health promotion and screening. It aims to give an account of the screening programmes currently available to all ages in the UK. The national screening programme does not screen for all diseases, however, and nurses need to be aware of this.

Health promotion and health screening

The role of health promotion in secondary prevention of ill health is to raise awareness of screening programmes available, to encourage people to attend and take up the invitations extended to them, and to support and help with understanding the results of the screening. Or, it may be that people need to be encouraged to go for testing at the first sign of a health problem. By finding out if a disease is present at an early stage, appropriate early treatment can make a successful outcome more likely. Secondary prevention involves action to seek out disease at an early stage followed by intervention during the early stages of the disease to prevent further damage. The action that is carried out is screening, allowing for treatment to commence at much earlier stages.

Concept summary: Disease prevention is at three levels

Primary prevention
Action to keep people healthy and free from disease, for example, encouragement of healthy lifestyle or immunisation.

Secondary prevention
Action to identify disease in people, which they can be unaware of, for example, screening.

Tertiary prevention
Actions taken to promote recovery or prevent further disability once a disease has developed, for example, rehabilitation, advice on the use of medicines, advice on lifestyle changes, and support to live well with the disease.

Screening therefore has the potential to save lives, or improve the quality of life, by the process of early detection or diagnosis of serious conditions and encouraging people to seek treatment at the first sign of a health problem.

It is not a foolproof process. However, screening reduces the risk of development or further development of an existing condition (which may have complications), but it cannot give guarantees of protection. Not all health issues are suitable for screening. Any decision to develop large-scale screening programmes will involve collecting a great deal of medical evidence and consideration of the ethical issues. Health promotion must also include an advocacy function, to encourage informed public debate and discussion as policies evolve for large-scale screening programmes.

There are occasions in any screening programme where there will be a number of results wrongly reporting some people as having the condition. These are referred to as false positives and wrong reports of not having the condition are called false negatives. It is important that there are realistic expectations of what a screening programme has to offer. The UK National Screening Committee (UK NSC) is increasingly presenting screening as risk reduction, not risk elimination, thus emphasising the limitations (UK NSC, 2015). Screening can reduce the risk of developing a condition or the complications of that condition. However, it cannot offer guarantees of protection.

National screening programmes

The UK NSC and NHS screening programmes are a part of Public Health England, an executive agency of the Department of Health. The UK NSC advises ministers and the NHS in the four UK countries about all aspects of screening, collating research evidence and regularly reviewing policy on screening. The UK NSC makes the UK-wide policies but it is up to the different parts of the UK to decide how and when the policies are set up in practice. This will mean that there may be some differences in the services available depending on whether you live in England, Scotland, Wales or Northern Ireland. In the UK, there is screening for a range of health problems and conditions throughout life, from antenatal and newborn screening programmes, with testing carried out at set times, to childhood, mid-life and later-life screening. As a nurse you may not find yourself directly involved in practice with patients undergoing all the screening tests, but you must know enough to understand and answer patients' questions.

Antenatal and newborn screening

NHS antenatal screening includes ultrasound imaging, and tests for Down's syndrome, sickle cell disease, thalassaemia, foetal anomaly, and infectious diseases (HIV, hepatitis B, syphilis and rubella). The screening programme aims to offer testing and information to all pregnant women. NHS newborn screening involves testing hearing, newborn physical examination and the blood spot programme. The blood spot programme in the UK will offer screening for congenital hypothyroidism (CHT), phenylketonuria (PKU), sickle cell disease disorders (SCD), cystic fibrosis (CF) and medium-chain acyl-CoA dehydrogenase deficiency (MCADD). For regional variations check the individual websites for Scotland, Northern Ireland, England and Wales.

The UK NSC Newborn Blood Spot Screening Programme in England from 2015 offers screening for four additional disorders. This screening is for maple syrup urine disease (MSUD), homocystinuria (HCU), isovaleric acidaemia (IVA) and glutaricaciduria type 1(GA1), and means that the screening programme in England offers screening for a total of nine disorders (UK NSC, 2015). Childhood screening continues with the school-entry health check, where three separate elements are checked at about four to five years of age. With parental consent, growth and height are monitored. An audiologist carries out a hearing assessment and an orthoptist will assess vision.

To get a good idea of the tests available for antenatal and newborn screening, consult the antenatal and newborn screening timeline optimum times for testing found at the UK NHS screening website (http://cpd.screening.nhs.uk/timeline).

Mid-life and later-life screening

For mid-life and later-life screening, national cancer screening programmes in the UK exist for breast, cervical and bowel cancer. Where screening for cancer is possible, it is a key tool in detecting abnormalities at early stages. This allows treatment to be started when the cancer has the best chance of being cured, or in some cases even before it develops. When considering cancer screening in the UK, it is important to remember that each country within the UK (England and Wales, Scotland and Northern Ireland) will each have their individual screening programmes. There may be slight differences in age ranges for invitation to attend the screening. It is useful to familiarise yourself (on the UK NSC website) with the various details for this wherever your geographical location. You may want to find what to expect in the area where you live and what will be happening where you are working in clinical practice. Make sure that you select the appropriate country. The UK NSC manages the specific programmes for cancer screening in the UK. It issues guidance on which screening programmes should be supported and also gives details on how to implement and monitor them (UK NSC, 2015).

Breast screening

Breast screening involves taking a mammogram of each breast (an X-ray of the carefully compressed breast). Potential patients may have a variety of concerns, both personal and cultural, about breast screening, so it is important to inform them that the staff at NHS breast screening units in the UK are women only. If a patient worries that the procedure sounds painful, reassure her that women who take up the screening test usually remark that it is quite uncomfortable but not painful. This may make a difference as to whether a woman will attend her screening appointment. The mammogram can detect small changes in breast tissue, which may be too small to feel on breast examination, for either the woman or her practice nurse. The invitation to attend breast screening in the UK is given to women aged between 50 and 70, every three years (women over the age of 70 are not sent invitations but are encouraged to make their own appointments). From 2012, the screening programme began extending in England to the ages of 47–73. This means that women can have the opportunity to have two extra screening invitations in their lifetime.

Breast screening pilot studies were set up to investigate the practicalities of inviting women aged 47–49 and 71–73 years in addition to the women in the 50–70 years age group. This age extension of the Breast Screening Programme started with a full randomised controlled trial in 2012 and full roll-out of the programme is expected to be completed after 2016. The age extension will be gradually phased in across England; this means that not everyone will be invited straight away.

Randomising the gradual extension of the screening allows for scientific evaluation, and researchers at Oxford University will analyse results on behalf of the NHS Breast Screening Programme.

∙∙∙

Case study: Extending breast screening in England

Mrs Papadopoulos is a 72-year-old lady who has received an invitation and appointment time to attend for a mammogram. She last attended a screening three years ago and thought that this would be her last invitation to attend screening, as she had read that the age range for mammograms in the NHS was 50–70 years. Included with the invitation is the leaflet 'Extending the Screening Age'.

This leaflet gives details about how breast screening is being extended at either end of the age range. Because Mrs Papadopoulos lives in an area where the age etension to the NHS breast screening has been introduced, she has been randomly selected to be invited for screening. This means she will have another screening beyond 70 years. Mrs Papadopoulos is delighted to be included in the new age extension to the screening programme. This means she will not have to make contact in this instance with her local screening unit to request a further appointment for screening beyond 70 years.

∙∙∙

Younger women with a family history of breast cancer will be offered regular screening and may also benefit from the addition of a different type of screening test with an MRI (magnetic resonance imaging) scan. This type of screening is found to be more sensitive for the dense breast tissue in younger women (Salem et al., 2013). Research to support screening in younger women with relatives with breast cancer has added to the debate to extend the screening programme further, thereby preventing deaths from cancer, suggesting specifically yearly screening for women aged 40–49 (Kopans, 2010).

MRI scans are not used routinely to screen women for breast cancer but NICE Excellence recommends the use of MRI in women under 40 who are at a very high risk (for example, women who have one of the breast cancer susceptibility genes) because MRI has been shown to be a more sensitive test than mammography in this group.

Starting in 2013, younger women at a high risk of developing breast cancer were incorporated into the NHS Breast Screening Programme. They have an MRI scan as well as mammograms; the exact type of managing surveillance will depend on their individual type of risk. These women fall into two groups: (1) a strong family history of breast or othersite cancer, having been assessed by geneticists and (2) women who have had radiotherapy to the chest for lymphoma or leukaemia when under the age of 25. Women at a moderate risk and low increased risk are managed under locally arranged surveillance and self-awareness protocols.

A study reported in the *Journal of the Royal Society of Medicine* (Mukhtar et al., 2013) suggested that breast cancer screening may not have reduced deaths from the disease and questioned the role of mammography. The study analysed death rates in breast cancer in the Oxford region, before and after the introduction of the UK's NHS Breast Screening Programme in 1988. The study reported that the greatest reduction in breast cancer deaths was in women under 40 years of age. However, this is an age group that has not routinely been offered screening. This study runs counter to the results of other studies. The Marmot Report (Marmot et al., 2013) reported a 20 per cent relative reduction in breast cancer deaths in women offered screening and concluded that breast screening saves lives. In addition, the Oxford study has been criticised. The senior director of cancer screening at the American Cancer Society, Robert Smith, cited flaws in the statistical method used in the study and referred to an earlier study that he had completed with colleagues (Duffy et al., 2010), where they reported that the benefit in terms of lives saved is greater than the harm of over-diagnosis and that there are more studies that show the benefit of screening than those that do not. The media coverage of such reports about breast screening may alarm or confuse women and you may find them anxious to discuss matters with you, their nurse. You need to be aware of the issues raised.

Encouraging women to be aware of their breasts, that is, to know what they look and feel like at different times, should assist women to understand what is normal for them and therefore detect any unusual changes. This approach is supported by the *Be Breast Aware* leaflet produced by the NHS Breast Screening Programme and Cancer Research UK, published in 2008 and available at www.gov.uk in 18 languages. The Department of Health's policy on breast awareness, supported strongly by the nursing and medical professions, does not advocate routine self-examination to a set technique, but does encourage women to check their breasts and know what is normal for them, and therefore know when changes occur. The scientific evidence to support formal, ritual self-examination, performed at the same time each month, is lacking. Instead, the NHS Breast Screening Programme sets out a five-point plan:

- know what is normal for you;

- look and feel;

- know what changes to look for;

- report changes without delay;

- attend breast screening when invited.

It may be useful to be aware of the fact that some women in the UK will consult American websites about breast examination. They will find that the ritual of routine self-examination, to a set technique, at a set time each month, is still encouraged in that country. This may cause confusion, but careful direction to the NHS Breast Screening Programme and the Cancer Research UK five-point plan should give clarification. You may wish to get your own copy of the five-point plan to familiarise yourself with the guidelines, so that you can have a well-informed discussion with any patient who may raise this issue.

Activity 3.1   *Communication*

A woman approaches you in your clinic and asks for advice. She is puzzled about the Breast Screening Programme as she has reached her fiftieth birthday and has not yet been sent her invitation to attend a screening unit for a mammogram. She is worried that she has been left out and is confused as her friend, who is 48, has received an invitation to attend.

- What response do you offer her?

An outline answer is provided at the end of the chapter.

More people in the UK are aware of breast cancer in women due to strong and repeated health promotion campaigns. People shopping in high street pharmacies or clothing stores will be familiar with Breast Cancer Awareness Month in October each year and will find pink ribbon lapel badges on sale to raise funds for cancer research. Many people are unaware, however, of the fact that men can also develop breast cancer. Men have a small amount of breast tissue behind each nipple and it is here that the breast cancer can develop. Breast cancer in men is rare and there is no screening programme. In the UK around 378 men are diagnosed each year and, like women, the single biggest risk is age. Most cases are diagnosed between the ages of 60 and 70 (Cancer Research UK, 2014a)

Male patients are disadvantaged by a lack of research and there are important biological differences between male and female breast cancer. Male patients are more likely to be diagnosed later than female patients. New research in the Netherlands has found some of the biological differences between male and female types of breast cancer and it is hoped that this will make better treatment choices for male patients (ECCO, 2016).

Recently, within the UK, there have been some awareness-raising campaigns for improving breast cancer screening programmes for black women. The argument is that, for many years, the 'face' for women's breast cancer has been the white middle-class woman who features in posters and advertisements raising awareness. Lack of a wider range of ethnic images adds to the perception that other groups of women are not at such risk of developing breast cancer. This has led to women being diagnosed late and inequalities in survival rates. Evidence for this has come from a small UK study (Bowen et al., 2008) with more studies carried out in the USA on African American women. These studies demonstrated that black women develop breast cancer, on average, 10 to 20 years younger than white women. Black women were less at risk of developing breast cancer but, for those who did, it had a tendency to be a more aggressive type of breast cancer. This has implications for the screening age set currently at 50 for some women, with extension to 47 years in England from 2012, as this is too high a starting age for black women. Ensuring that black women have a greater awareness of the signs and symptoms of breast cancer, and improving their access and uptake of breast screening, has been the subject of research by Betterdays Cancer Care, in southeast London.

Known as the Patient Navigation Project, it was based on and adapted from a US public health initiative where people (patient navigators) from the same cultural background guide patients through the healthcare system. Acting as supporters, they raised awareness and helped overcome barriers to accessing services. Southwark and Lewisham in London were selected for the pilot project, as uptake of screening for both black and ethnic minority groups living there is lower than the national average. The Patient Navigation Project concluded it was effective in engaging with women who would not have otherwise had their breast screening (mammography) and raised awareness among the community (Betterdays Cancer Care, 2012).

A further group of women who will need increased awareness about breast cancer are British South Asian women. Researchers in Sheffield concluded, after a study conducted in Leicester, that the historic picture of low risk of disease among this group of women is no longer the case (Day, 2013). Between 2000 and 2004, South Asian women had a 45 per cent lower rate of breast cancer compared with white women. By 2005–9, however, breast cancer rates increased in South Asian women, to be 8 per cent higher than in the population of white women, whose rates did not show significant change. The change was statistically significant for the 65-year age group of South Asian women, at 37 per cent higher than white women. The Breakthrough Breast Cancer Charity has requested further research to see if the trend is also true for South Asian women across the UK, to understand the reasons behind this change.

Case study: Learning disability and breast cancer screening

Fiona acts as carer for her sister, Rosie, who is aged 52 and has learning disabilities. Fiona is concerned when a letter arrives inviting Rosie to attend a mammography appointment, as part of the local breast screening programme. Fiona wonders how she should proceed with this appointment for Rosie, who lacks the mental capacity to make her own decisions about screening. Following consultation with Rosie's practice nurse she learns that she may make a 'best interest' decision. That is, she makes a decision on behalf of Rosie in the same way that she makes decisions about other aspects of Rosie's care and treatment. Whether a person is a paid carer, unpaid family member or close friend, the process is the same. The practice nurse tells Fiona of a publication about making best interest decisions that she feels will give her clear information (Office of the Public Guardian, 2009). She also reminds Fiona that staff at the NHS mobile screening unit are all women (Rosie will find this acceptable) and that she can phone the radiographer in advance to let them know about Rosie. Together they agree that Rosie, if possible, should have the mammogram as their mother had breast cancer.

A useful resource with accessible health information, using words and pictures, can be found at www.easyhealth.org.uk

Cervical screening

Cervical screening is not a test for cancer. It is, however, a test to check the health of the cells of the cervix (previously known as a smear test) and takes a sample of cells from a woman's cervix using a special brush; a practice nurse or doctor does this test. A cytologist carefully examines the sample. By detection of any abnormal cells and commencing early treatment, it prevents cancer of the cervix developing. All four UK countries now offer Human Papilloma Virus (HPV) testing. Certain kinds of HPV can cause abnormal cell changes in the cervix and, if they are left untreated, these abnormal cells may go on to develop cervical cancer. If a sample taken at the cervical screening test has a low grade abnormality, the sample cells are automatically tested for HPV. If HPV is found then the woman is referred for a colposcopy for further investigation and treatment. In all four UK countries women in the age range 25–49 years are invited every three years for cervical screening. Women in the age range 50–64 are invited for screening every five years. Cervical cancer is very rare in women under 25 years (Landy et al., 2014).

Activity 3.2   *Communication*

A family friend approaches you for advice, as she knows you are a nurse. She is 25 years old and has received a letter calling her for a cervical screening test (cervical smear), but she tells you that she has not been sexually active since she was at college. She thinks that she needn't bother with the test but wants to be sure that she is correct.

- What is your response?

An outline answer is provided at the end of the chapter.

Research (Gok et al., 2010) indicates that the availability of self-sampling test kits to detect the HPV in women would increase screening. The HPV can cause damage to cervical cells and this may develop into cervical cancer. It is suggested that this method of collecting cervico-vaginal specimens is an effective way of increasing coverage in a screening programme. The NHS is piloting research for this testing as an 'add-on' to traditional screening, as not all younger women take up the invitation for cervical smear testing. The researchers believe that this form of screening could double the number of women diagnosed with the HPV, as women are more likely to carry out self-testing at home. Non-attendance to smear test screening, particularly among younger women, is a major concern in the effectiveness of current cervical screening programmes in the UK. The data suggest that one woman in five does not attend appointments sent out to them (Weller and Campbell, 2009). A further study has explored the various reasons for women not attending cervical screening, particularly in the 25–29 age group in England. It was identified that there were barriers in all age groups. Older women had a negative attitude to screening, younger women intended to be screened but did not attend (Waller et al., 2012). (See Chapter 6 for information on HPV vaccines for 12–13-year-old girls in the UK.)

Ovarian cancer screening

Currently there is no screening programme for ovarian cancer. However, one of the largest ever randomised controlled trials suggested screening could reduce mortality by 20 per cent. A simple blood test is used for testing for the CA 125 protein (cancer antigen 125). CA 125 is produced by some ovarian cancer cells. UK researchers studied more than 200,000 women recruited from centres in England, Wales and Northern Ireland between 2001 and 2005, and followed up for an average of 11 years. Women were aged between 50 and 74 years. The authors of the study say further follow-up is needed to determine whether routine screening of the general population would be cost effective, but that this study opens up a new discussion in the quest for ovarian cancer research and care (Jacobs et al., 2015). The UK National Screening Committee will be monitoring the futher data collected to see if screening would be a good use of NHS resources.

Bowel cancer screening

Bowel cancer screening aims to detect cancer at early stages in symptom-free people, when treatment is likely to be effective. The NHS offers bowel screening with a bowel scope to men and women starting at 55 years of age in England. Bowel screening using a bowel scope or flexiscope is a fairly new test. The flexiscope is placed in the rectum and lower bowel and allows an illuminated examination. If any small growths called polyps (growths found on mucosal surfaces) are found then they can be removed as they could possibly turn into cancer. The programme is gradually being rolled out to men and women in England. Depending on where you are in practice, it may not yet be offered to your patients. For every 300 people screened it can prevent two from getting bowel cancer and saves one life from bowel cancer. The flexiscope screening of the bowel is a once-only test and patients will receive an invitation to attend their local screening centre. The flexiscope screening occurred as a result of a 16 year clinical trial cofunded by Cancer Research UK (Cancer Research UK, 2010) and the research was conducted in 14 centres (Atkin et al., 2010). As from March 2015 about two thirds of screening centres are beginning to offer the test to 55-year-olds. The original goal of all screening centres to be offering this screening by 2016 has not been achieved.

Training nurse endoscopists already occurs in many centres and it would be expected that training opportunities will increase to meet clinical needs. Patients will have the test offered up until the age of 60 years when they will be transferred to the other screening system. From 60 years onwards, screening involves participants being sent a postal test kit for faecal occult blood (FOB) so that, in the privacy of their own home, they can carry out three stool tests. Clear guidelines as to how to complete the tests are provided in an instruction leaflet. The completed test kit is then posted in a special envelope provided to a regional laboratory for analysis. Any man or woman with a positive result will be invited for colonoscopy to see if polyps or cancer are present. The testing kit is automatically sent out to patients in the post and the test is carried out every two years. The age range for the FOB testing is 60–74 years in England, Wales and Northern Ireland. Scotland offers the FOB test from 50–74 years.

Activity 3.3   *Communication*

A neighbour approaches you as she knows you are a nurse. She has found out that she is under the age set for bowel cancer screening, but she is worried as her sister had bowel cancer two years ago. She confides that she has symptoms of a change in bowel habits and asks you if she should be asking to be tested.

• What is your response?

An outline answer is provided at the end of the chapter.

Case study: Bowel cancer screening – the need to confirm understanding in those requiring assistance

Cynthia is a community nurse involved in the team of carers looking after 65-year-old Mrs Begum in her own home. Mrs Begum uses a wheelchair and requires assistance with hygiene needs. One morning Cynthia arrives to find that Mrs B has received a bowel screening kit in the post and she shows this to

(continued)

continued . . .

Cynthia. They look together at the instructions for sample collecting in the guidelines that accompany the test kit. Cynthia takes note of the fact that Mrs Begum has a good understanding of what the bowel screening is offering; she understands about the three stool samples for faecal occult blood (FOB). Further, Cynthia also takes note of the fact that Mrs Begum has a full understanding of what a colonoscopy examination entails. On the basis of this comprehensive understanding, when Mrs Begum asks Cynthia if she can have assistance in completing the tests in the kit, Cynthia agrees. She knows that Mrs Begum has the mental capacity to consent to the screening.

Prostate Cancer Risk Management Programme

Currently there is no screening programme for prostate cancer (Cancer Research UK, 2014b). A screening programme would need to have a test that would reliably find cancer during a man's lifetime. There is a test called the PSA test (Prostate Specific Antigen), which can help doctors work out how likely a man is to have prostate cancer. However, this test is not reliable enough to provide a national screening programme and there is no clear evidence to support the idea that using the PSA test could save lives. The prostate gland is found in men below the bladder and surrounding the urethra. PSA is a protein produced by prostate cells and it can be measured by a blood test. PSA levels can be raised if a man has prostate cancer. However, the levels can also be raised when a man has other conditions that are not cancer, such as an enlarged prostate. It is difficult to say what is a normal level and what is high as all men have slightly different PSA levels.

Men over the age of 50 can ask their GP for a PSA blood test and this is part of the UK Prostate Cancer Risk Management Programme. The GP will explain about all the benefits and risks and give patients written information to read. Men under the age of 50 are considered low risk. The IMPACT trial started in 2005 and is due to run until the end of 2016. It is studying men who have a faulty gene and therefore have an increased risk of developing prostate cancer (Cancer Research UK, 2014c). IMPACT stands for **I**dentification of **M**en with a genetic predisposition to **P**rost**A**te cancer: **T**argeted screening in men at higher genetic risk and controls (Cancer Research UK, 2014c).

Activity 3.4   *Communication*

A gentleman approaches you in an outpatients' clinic and tells you that his wife has read in the newspaper about a special test for men to check for prostate cancer. He wonders if this is correct and, if so, whether it would be appropriate for him to have the test, as his father had prostate cancer.

- What is your response?

An outline answer is provided at the end of the chapter.

There are some other types of screening described later in the chapter, but first we will discuss how to encourage more people to attend screening programmes.

Uptake of UK screening services

Methods employed to encourage the uptake of screening services are set out in a report by Cancer Research UK (2008). It is useful to consider these initiatives or actions, as this should increase your understanding of how and why NHS screening may or may not have a 'good' uptake where you live or where you work in clinical practice. The report lists seven initiatives or areas of good practice.

Research summary: Good practice in screening services

- **Joint working**: The idea is to ensure that the same messages get put across about the screening programmes available and that best use is made of staff expertise and equipment. Joint working also includes awareness-raising campaigns, for example to encourage the use of the screening services and remove barriers to understanding in certain population areas. The report identifies local community health organisations working along with other organisations. For example, this could be neighbouring community health organisations, hospital trusts, and private and voluntary sectors.
- **Public campaigns and health promotion**: The report gives examples of media campaigns to raise awareness, particularly targeting ethnic communities with low uptake.
- **Targeting community initiatives**: This might be a specific geographical area that is a community or it might be a specific age group of people who would be focused on for screening.
- **Working within GP practices**: The report highlights the usefulness of, for example, in-surgery poster displays and links with local pharmacies.
- **Service improvements**: This means providing extra locations for screening facilities and extending the hours, sometimes giving a choice of attending different locations, again focusing on a particular target group.
- **Equity audits and research**: This is about the gathering of information about certain groups in the population, to identify low uptake, to have future specific targeting and to gain better understanding of uptake.
- **Screening databases**: This is not a direct method of improving uptake of screening. However, improved, updated databases of current eligible individuals would have an impact on those populations offered screening coverage. This is particularly important in mobile populations.

(Cancer Research UK, 2008)

The 'one size fits all' approach to health information is not appropriate in meeting the needs of the UK's increasingly diverse population and there is a constant need to find ways to target groups and communities that have a low uptake of screening services, in other words a variety of approaches. Health literacy (see Chapter 4) varies to a large extent in the population, and socio-economic status is a powerful driver of uptake of screening (Weller and Campbell, 2009). Within the UK there is a wide variation in uptake in cancer screening programmes among different populations or groups of people (read about health inequalities in Chapter 6).

To see how nurses might go about the business of behaviour change in relation to uptake of health screening, refer back to the section on behaviour change methods in Chapter 2 (pages 39–44).

Other types of screening

The following screening programmes are not all about cancer prevention. The screening is still about actions to improve health, and to test for hidden disease or disease at an early stage.

Diabetic retinopathy screening

The aim of this NHS screening programme is to prevent the risk of sight loss among people with diabetes, by identifying sight-threatening diabetic retinopathy (leaking blood vessels in the retina at the back of the eye), and to facilitate appropriate treatment.

The screening process involves digital photography of the retina. By grading the results, the eyes can be screened for signs of retinopathy. Screening is offered to people over 12 years of age with diabetes. All four UK countries have implemented diabetic retinopathy screening; look for details of individual country approaches in the UK.

Activity 3.5 *Communication*

A patient's daughter approaches you and asks for advice. You are a part of the team caring for her elderly mother (a respite care arrangement) and you know that the daughter is currently receiving treatment for her depression. She also has type 2 diabetes. Recently she received a letter asking her to attend for diabetic eye screening. She doesn't understand this, it makes her feel anxious and she feels there is not time to do this, as well as visit her mother.

- How do you respond to this situation?

An outline answer is provided at the end of the chapter.

The health check (vascular risk)

This NHS health check programme for vascular risk started in April 2009 and it targets everyone between the ages of 40 and 74 to prevent heart disease, stroke, diabetes and kidney disease. All people not already diagnosed with one of these conditions will be invited every five years to have a check to assess their risk and receive advice and support to help reduce or manage any risk. This was a phased programme, expecting full programme implementation by 2013. This disease management programme was crticised by a House of Commons report in 2014, which argued that the programme did not have a robust evidence base. The UK National Screening Committee, however, provided information about the programme (UK NSC, 2014). This health check is currently carried out at GP practices and some of these vascular checks will involve practice nurses. Posters displayed in surgeries promoting this service encourage and invite patients to make an appointment.

In England the responsibility for these health checks was transferred to local authorities in April 2013 and the checks will be commissioned from suitable providers.

NHS health screening for the over 65s

Some additional opportunities for health screening exist for people in the older age group, while there is a continuation of screening started in earlier adulthood. As people get older they are more likely to develop conditions that are rare in younger people. Men and women over 65 continue to be invited to bowel cancer screening until the age of 70. There are now plans to extend this age range further (see above). Over this age, people can continue to have screening by request. Breast cancer screening for women will continue up to age 70, with plans to extend this to 73 (see above). Requests by individuals can be made to local screening units to be included in the screening beyond this age. Women from the age of 65 no longer receive an invitation for cervical screening, unless they have had a previous abnormal screening result from any of the past three screening tests. Women who have never undertaken screening are entitled to ask for a test, regardless of age.

AAA screening

The NHS abdominal aortic aneurysm (AAA) programme (NHS, 2014) aims to reduce death from AAA through early detection. This programme is for men when they reach the age of 65 (over 65s may request this screening), who are offered an invitation to screening to measure the width of the aorta, involving a simple ultrasound scan of the abdomen. The aorta is the main blood vessel supplying blood to the body. In some people the wall of the aorta can, with age, become weak and start to swell, forming an aneurysm. The aim of this screening is to reduce the number of deaths related to this condition, most common in men aged 65 and over. The AAA screening programme was set up in England in 2009 and, since the end of 2013, it is now offered throughout the UK. In February 2016 guidance on the nurse specialist role for local services for AAA screening in England was published. Nurse specialists are described as experienced specialist vascular nurses. The background and training description for this role is included in the guidelines, along with details of how to provide assessment, support and lifestyle advice to the men in the screening programme (NHS, 2016).

Opportunistic screening

Screening can be considered to be 'opportunistic' when a test is carried out for a patient during a consultation for a completely different condition. The appointment has given an excellent opportunity to discuss other relevant health matters.

....
Case study: An example of opportunistic screening

A middle-aged man comes to the general practice where you are on placement. He has backache. The records state that he last attended the practice five years ago. Following the back pain consultation, the GP refers him straight away to the practice nurse for blood pressure testing. The practice nurse is coordinating vascular risk screening in the practice. Here is a chance to obtain a measurement of his blood pressure. The only way of knowing if an individual has high blood pressure is to have it measured. Many people who have high blood pressure have no symptoms at all; as a result it can often go undiagnosed (British Heart Foundation, 2015). One in every three adults and just over three in ten men have high blood pressure.
....

The National Chlamydia Screening Programme

Clamydia is a sexually transmitted bacterial infection that affects around 2–3 per cent of sexually active young adults. Untreated it can have serious consequences, including pelvic inflammatory disease (PID) which can lead to ectopic pregnancy and infertility in women. Men can develop epididymitis (swelling of the tubes in the testicles). However, chlamydia is easy to diagnose and treat. The national chlamydia screening programme recommends that all sexually active men and women aged 15–24 be tested for chlamydia annually or on change of sexual partner (whichever is more frequent). Chlamydia screening is an effective way to deliver good health promotion messages and has been found to be widely acceptable. Giving information and support ensures young people have knowledge and become empowered to protect themselves from sexually transmitted infections (STI). Screening can be delivered opportunistically. Sexually active young adults should be offered a test when attending community sexual and reproductive services, pharmacies or GPs. In addition, service can also be provided through self-sampling kits. Until 2013 the responsibility for sexual and reproductive health services came under Primary Care Trusts but this responsibility was then transferred to local authorities (LAs). Local authorities have since been building on the progress in addressing chlamydia through screening by ensuring that access is easy for young adults and ensuring good quality opportunistic screening. A quick way to find out about the screening in your local area is to visit the Public Health Outcomes Framework website and view the list of health indicators for local authorities.

Community nurses can have a particular role in chlamydia screening, working in GP practices. Education events such as health fairs are often held in colleges and universities and can raise awareness about chlamydia, offering and encouraging participants to take up screening and giving out test kits, which can then be completed in private by the young people. The test kit comprises either a urine test for men or a vaginal swab (like a tampon) for women. After the test is completed the kit can either be posted to the testing laboratory direct or handed back to the community nurse, who then forwards all kits for analysis. The participant is then contacted with the result and, if positive, he or she will be prescribed a course of antibiotics.

Screening new patients at GP practices

As well as the screening programmes mentioned above, there are many tests that people may expect to be carried out by their GP and they include the 'new patient health check', where selected tests are carried out as part of this routine screening. This involves measuring height and weight, checking up on current vaccination status, general health, diet and physical activity advice, urinalysis testing and blood pressure testing. The British Hypertension Society advises that all adults have a blood pressure check every five years, or every year if they are over 75 or if they have high blood pressure (Williams et al., 2004).

Occupational health screening

Occupational health is concerned with the health and welfare of people engaged in work or employment. It actively promotes the maintenance of good health in the workplace and supports employers and employees when health problems occur. The aim of screening for occupational health is to advise managers on prospective employees' fitness for job requirements. This advice would be given where necessary, on any adjustments to work content or environment that might be needed, in view of any disability in line with the Equality Act of 2010, and to identify any work-related health risks of future employment. A health screening programme will help detect disease or risk factors early so that further progression can be stopped or the outcome improved. The three elements to the screening are as follows.

- Completion of a full health questionnaire. There may be a consultation with the prospective employee's GP. Occupational health screening may stop at this point if all is satisfactory.

- Further assessment, if necessary, following completion of the questionnaire, will involve offering a clinic appointment with the occupational health service department, to ascertain fitness to work.

- Immunisation where recommended, at the beginning of employment, will be arranged by and administered by the occupational health service.

At this point you may think back to the occupational health screening that you undertook as you commenced your own nursing education programme. You will probably now understand better the process of assessment of your fitness for practice in the clinical settings, and the risk detection offered by screening.

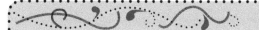

Chapter summary

This chapter has raised your awareness of large-scale national screening programmes available in four UK countries and their contribution to health and well-being for patients. It has outlined the range of screening that individuals could expect to experience during their lifespan. Patients often turn to their nurses for clarification and explanation of matters relating to health, so it is important that nurses are well informed about the role of health promotion and raising awareness about screening. Nurses can encourage and support patients as they accept invitations to take part in screening, which has the potential to save lives or improve the quality of life. Health promotion must have an advocacy function, which includes the encouragement of informed debate and discussion, as new evidence and policy emerges for extended or new large-scale screening programmes. Nurses need to be aware of these.

Activities: brief outline answers

Activity 3.1: Communication (page 55)

The friend of this woman has been invited as part of the age extension in England for screening, which includes the 47–49 and 71–73 age groups. The GP practice that she is registered with has been included in the age extension screening. The 50-year-old woman in your clinic lives in an area where the extension has not yet begun, so she will not be screened before the first routine invitation, which will arrive before her 53rd birthday.

Explain that the screening is a rolling programme, that is, a system that calls women from their GP practices in turn. The invitation arrives at some time between the age of 50 and 53. Women are automatically sent this if they are registered with a GP.

It is good to advise patients to keep their GP practice up to date with correct contact details. You can reassure the woman by informing her that she could get in touch with her practice and ask to speak to the practice nurse. She can then ask when the practice is on the schedule for their screening to be carried out and so can calculate roughly when she is likely to be sent her invitation.

Activity 3.2: Communication (page 58)

You should explain the facts to your family friend so that she can make her decision about her health screening. There is evidence to show that, if a woman has never been sexually active, her risk of developing cervical cancer is extremely low. The language used here is not 'no risk' but 'low risk'.

If a woman has ever had sex she will probably have come into contact with the human papilloma virus (HPV), which causes cervical cancer. The evidence suggests, therefore, that it is appropriate to accept the appointment and have the cervical smear test. She may like to contact her practice nurse, who will carry out the test and explain to her what exactly is involved.

Activity 3.3: Communication (page 59)

Your response must be that it is unwise for your neighbour to wait for screening in this instance. Persistent change in bowel habits or anxiety about bowel health in general should be investigated. Your neighbour must be encouraged to seek medical advice urgently and consult her GP, who could arrange for referral to a specialist if necessary, in view of her family history.

Activity 3.4: Communication (page 60)

Your reply should confirm to this man that his wife would have read about the prostate testing offered to men aged 50 and over.

Are some men more at risk of developing prostate cancer? The biggest risk factor is age and other factors include a family history of the disease. In the UK risk is also greater in black Caribbean and black African men. His question about his father could be significant, especially if this prostate cancer occurred before the age of 60.

It is important that men receive the best available information and support. This man needs to be given a written information sheet from his practice, which fully explains what is involved in the test. He will also need to have a consultation with his GP. If he goes ahead with the test he will need to understand that this will involve having a blood test. The PSA (prostate-specific antigen) levels in the blood are measured.

This substance, made by the prostate gland, naturally leaks into the bloodstream. A raised level can be an early indication of prostate cancer. However, prostatitis, enlargement of the prostate and urinary infection can also cause a rise in PSA.

Activity 3.5: Communication (page 62)

This woman needs to have you spend time with her to discuss the letter, to reduce her anxiety and agitation. You can help explain to her the background or context to the screening invitation, which should help her concentration and overcome any feeling of helplessness she might have. If she has difficulty remembering things, suggest you can help her to write some notes she would find helpful.

It is important to screen for diabetic retinopathy to detect any changes in her retina at an early stage before she might be aware of them. Even if she attends an optometrist (optician), she needs to know that this is a specialist screening service. She must still attend her yearly appointment with her optometrist for her free sight checks for glasses. Suggest that she could take a friend with her. The screening test is painless, involving photographs of the back of each eye. She may have drops to dilate her pupils, making her vision a bit blurry for a while, so it would be helpful to have an escort, and she must not drive until her vision recovers.

Reassure her that you can help to explain to her mother the importance of keeping the appointment and explain and remind her mother about the temporary absence of the daughter.

Useful websites

https://www.gov.uk/topic/population-screening-programmes

This useful link lists the population screening programmes available in the UK, find out about them here.

www.cancerresearch.org

There is a wide range of information about cancer screening and campaigns on this cancer research institute site.

https://www.gov.uk/guidance/prostate-cancer-risk-management-programme-overview

Here you will find an overview of the prostate cancer risk management programme.

https://www.gov.uk/government/publications/nhs-breast-screening-awareness-leaflet

Look for the 'Be Breast Aware' leaflet available in 18 languages.

https://www.gov.uk/government/collections/breast-screening-information-leaflets

Look for breast screening information leaflets, find out about good practice, age extension trial and high-risk women.

https://www.gov.uk/government/statistics/national-chlamydia-screening-programme-ncsp-data-tables

Useful information about the national programme for chlamydia screening.

http://www.senseaboutscience.org/resources.php/7/making-sense-of-screening

Visit this charity website and look for the booklet about screening to weigh up the benefits and harms of health screening programmes.

Chapter 4
Teaching patients

Introduction

Case study: A poor teaching environment

Mrs Shah is accompanied by her husband to the eye clinic in the outpatients' department. She is temporarily using a wheelchair for mobility problems – she sprained her ankle very badly last week. Mrs Shah has just attended her first appointment with the ophthalmologist; she was referred by her GP and optometrist as she had persistent raised intraocular pressure in both eyes. They suspect that she may have the beginnings of glaucoma. She could experience loss of field of vision due to the raised pressure inside the eye pressing on the optic nerve if the glaucoma is left untreated. The ophthalmologist has ordered a visual field test today and prescribed eye drops, and wants to review her next week in the clinic. She is to see the nurse next; she finds the staff nurse friendly but is disappointed when she finds the conversation directed to Mr Shah about the eye drop regime. She is passive when Mr Shah is taught how to put the drops in. Mrs Shah also notices that the nurse had not asked her if she understands the significance of eye drop therapy or of raised intraocular pressure. She knows about glaucoma as her mother had the condition. That is why she has been so careful to attend for testing at the optometrist from her fortieth birthday as advised. A large part of the outpatient experience has been a disappointing one for Mrs Shah, as she feels unacknowledged and not encouraged to ask questions of the staff nurse about her eye health.

Nurses are expected to engage in good communication skills and, whether working in hospital or community settings, all nurses have the responsibility of carrying out health teaching with their patients. This role has to be considered carefully, providing information that is clear, accurate and meaningful. This will mean that nurses must engage with the various elements and aspects of being an approachable and effective teacher of health. The NHS National Quality Board (NQB) (DH, 2011) has agreed on a guide to the measurement of patient experience across the NHS. This framework includes: information, communication and education on clinical status, and progress and processes of care in order to facilitate autonomy, self-care and health promotion.

The staff nurse in the case study above has not asked Mrs Shah about what she knows and what she might further understand. There has not been relevant preparation of a good environment for this teaching. This chapter will consider what it means to be a good teacher of health and will help you understand why and how the staff nurse went wrong. It will look first at where teaching should be carried out, and then look at how people learn, considering barriers to learning. The chapter also helps you to think about how to plan learning, what methods you might use to teach and finally how to evaluate your teaching.

Where to carry out teaching

Nurses need to think carefully about where their teaching time with patients will be spent. The setting might be general practice, an outpatient clinic, a hospital or the patient's home. Finding a suitable location within the setting is important. Planning ahead if possible for privacy and uninterrupted time must be given particular thought, and the possible inclusion of partners, husbands, wives, a parent or carers as part of the teaching session, if appropriate. Alongside the careful choice of space and surroundings within the setting, to carry out teaching nurses must consider the level of motivation that their patients may or may not have. The role of the nurse in carrying out teaching is therefore to be as practical and realistic as possible, and to recognise the circumstances and need of each individual patient. There is a need to plan your teaching to take into account the distinctive requirements of patients. For example, some patients may find it difficult to say what it is they want to learn in terms of understanding what they need to know about their health. The reasons for this might be embarrassment, lack of familiarity with medical or technical terminology, denial of illness, pain or a disempowering feeling that the professionals know best.

How to carry out teaching and readiness to learn

When talking to people about health matters, nurses need to avoid using jargon or technical language, which may confuse or alienate. By introducing some structure to the teaching, patients will be able to absorb the information and nurses can facilitate deep learning (understanding) as opposed to just memorising (surface learning). By this we mean that nurses need to find out what patients already know and understand, and then proceed from this point. The nurse in the case study failed to consider this important issue and thus failed to provide a suitable teaching session for the patient, Mrs Shah. The next step would be to clarify and explain any unknown technical terms. This should help with future communications and could be useful when patients have discussions with other healthcare professionals. This structured approach to teaching should help start a partnership in communication. Additional points to consider are that there may be a limit to patients' memory capacity. Dividing the information into small amounts for teaching on more than one session may be useful, rather than packing all the information into one long session.

Barriers to learning

Patients are not always ready to learn, or indeed willing to learn. Judging a patient's ability to absorb your teaching is an important first step. Your aim may be to empower the patient by giving him or her all the necessary information as you feel this is so vital. However, you must first think about what could cause barriers to this process.

Activity 4.1   *Reflection*

Think back to an occasion on which you observed a patient being taught. Did you notice that she or he was not listening, or was saying she or he had had enough? Consider what was going on for that patient at the time.

- Could there have been internal physical barriers such as pain or tiredness?
- Could there have been internal emotional barriers such as distress, fear or depression?
- Perhaps the patient was unable to understand because she or he did not have the intellectual capacity – too young, poor memory or not well-educated.
- Was there anything in the external environment interfering with learning, such as noise, distractions or cold?
- Could it be the content of the session or the way the nurse taught, such as with too much jargon, too fast or not well explained? Perhaps the nurse did not look interested, or did not understand the topic herself.

Further guidance on this activity is provided at the end of the chapter.

Having looked at possible barriers to learning, you can now appreciate more how complex teaching patients can be. On one hand, patients are not always in a position to receive nurses' carefully planned teaching. On the other hand, you will meet patients eager and ready to learn, sometimes asking you questions before you are prepared.

How people learn

People tend to learn in similar ways when ready. You will remember learning new things yourself; how you struggled with new terminology and perhaps took time to grasp why there are several ways of thinking and doing in nursing, when you couldn't see the difference as yet. A theory that may help you think of levels of learning is that of Bloom (1984), who used a taxonomy of knowledge, comprehension, application, analysis, synthesis and evaluation. Some educationalists have more recently revised Bloom's work to use more active language – remembering, understanding, applying, analysing, creating and evaluating – and have reversed the top two categories as it seems that creativity may be a higher skill than evaluation. See the work of Anderson and Krathwohl on nwlink.com/~donclark/hrd/bloom.html.

Concept summary: Bloom's taxonomy, revised by Anderson and Krathwohl

Bloom's taxonomy (or levels) of learning (1984) explains how people build up from basic knowledge to being able to use that knowledge to make judgements about a topic – to 'know' it so well that they can decide on its worth.

- **Remembering**: recalling previously learned information, facts and principles. What is it?
- **Understanding**: comprehending and interpreting that knowledge, without seeing the implications yet. What does it mean?
- **Applying**: seeing the use for something, perhaps in a new situation, and how it fits in with a theory or practice in real life. How do I use it?
- **Analysing**: breaking down into parts, recognising connections and differences. Making inferences from facts. What does it consist of?
- **Evaluating**: making judgements about the values of things, measuring them against criteria of appraisal. Is it a good thing?
- **Creating**: putting things together to make a whole in a new way of thinking. Making a proposal or a plan. How does it come together as a whole?

You can use these levels to decide how much you want the patient to learn and how much you can teach him or her at any one time, for example in a series of sessions. It is probably enough in the first short session for the patient to know and understand his or her new diagnosis. Having reflected on that level, next time you could discuss how it will affect the person's daily life and, later, what choices the patient has in the management of his or her diagnosis.

Scenario: Bloom's taxonomy in practice

Mrs Carter is about to have an abdominal hysterectomy and first needs to recall the medical terminology that has been used in her consultations so far (Remembering), so that the words being used become familiar to her. She then needs to comprehend (Understanding) what this means, perhaps in terms of 'removal of my womb'. Ask her to explain it to you. Thinking what this means for her (Applying), she needs to know that this will stop her menstruation.

Bloom's three higher levels of learning go further, although Mrs Carter says to the nurse teaching her, 'That's all I need to know, thank you'. You could perhaps leave the rest for another time.

Next day she asks the nurse to explain how the surgery will be done – will she have stitches, and where, and what exactly will be removed? She's thinking of the details (Analysing). Following this level of learning a person gains insight into the idea and makes judgements about her choices (Evaluating) and Mrs Carter realises that this will be major surgery. She will need to be in hospital for a few days and she will need to rest and not take strenuous exercise for a few weeks. She begins to ask when she

continued . . .

can go home and manage her toddler son. Until now she has not thought to ask if she will go through the menopause. Finally, an overall appraisal of the interruption to her life is possible (Creating); now she is 'qualified' to make an informed choice to go ahead and she has the in-depth learning to make a plan for the future, free from the influence of fear of the unknown, or persuasion from others.

Recognise that this theory also applies to you learning nursing and, while you are reading this book, it also applies to your learning how to teach patients.

Planning teaching

Consider how often you have sat in teaching sessions and thought it was becoming hard to concentrate for that length of time. You are well and ready to learn. A patient may be able to concentrate only for a much shorter time. Five or ten minutes is often enough time for a patient teaching session. Twenty minutes for a one-to-one session would be the maximum.

Teaching should, of course, begin when the patient is ready and asking questions, or you may see that he or she is getting better and needs to know more, well before he or she goes home, but do not think it has to be done all at once.

Case study: Planned teaching sessions

Steven Walker is a lead nurse in an acute coronary care unit. The unit has high- and medium-dependency areas and Steven would like to organise patient teaching for those who have had a myocardial infarction (heart attack).

He knows that some information is better given earlier if the patient is anxious to know what has happened and what is happening now, but not all the information can be given at once. He makes a plan of sessions to be delivered during every patient's average five-day stay in the unit. The plan can of course be modified as appropriate.

Having made his plan, Steven then sets about making each session much more detailed, with ideas for the information required.

It is a good idea to have some general teaching plans to be used for groups of similar patients like this. A plan incorporates nursing knowledge of what the patients need to know, and how much they can learn while in hospital in this case. Community nurses could use the same principle to design teaching plans for use in patients' homes. Each patient is different, of course, and the plan will have to be modified as it is implemented in practice. Some suggested modifications can be incorporated in the details, as Steven has done for men, women and elderly patients.

Detailed teaching materials need to be prepared by each clinical area and kept in a folder for use by nurses teaching the sessions. Steven has made a collection including a model and diagram of a heart, some printed material on healthy eating, explanations of the common drugs used, leaflets explaining the rehabilitation classes, and leaflets from the British Heart Foundation. Nurses using the teaching folder make sure that the material is up to date. In addition, the unit computer should be used to access information.

When using any teaching plan for a patient, whether pre-prepared or designed with the individual in mind, it is essential to begin with asking what the patient knows already. A good start to a teaching session would be to ask the patient what she or he knows about the topic of the session. You then know what to go over as a reminder, and what is new information for the patient.

Activity 4.2   *Communication*

Outline teaching plans for one of the following patients. Consider the variation in learning ability between them. Suggest some teaching resources to use.

- A boy of ten who needs to learn how to understand and use an inhaler when he has an asthma attack.
- A 28-year-old woman with a learning disability who was seen in casualty having poked a metal hair grip into her outer ear to clear wax. She has a superficial infection.
- A teenage boy with depression and self-neglect who needs to manage a course of oral antibiotics.
- An 82-year-old woman who has been diagnosed with non-insulin-dependent diabetes and says she doesn't understand why people are concerned about her feet.

An outline answer is provided at the end of the chapter.

You will have noticed some of the variables in learning ability in the patients from the last activity. Age and mental ability alter the level of learning that can be achieved, but nurses can address this through adapting their teaching to suit the patient's level. Guidance on teaching children and people with learning disabilities and altered mental states is not possible in detail here and we suggest you look at specialised books and relevant organisations for more information.

Teaching a skill

Some of your teaching will be about helping patients to acquire skills as well as knowledge. The activity above has the examples of using an inhaler and cleaning ears. You will meet patients who need to learn how to use equipment such as syringes and blood sugar monitors. Some patients need to know how to undertake procedures such as self-catheterisation and managing a feeding tube. Most of what the patient needs to know is what *you* have learned about the skill, with adaptations for using the equipment at home, not in hospital.

Activity 4.3 *Reflection*

Think of a single skill (practical procedure) you have acquired – a procedure or how to use a piece of equipment.

- How did you learn that skill? Recall methods of teaching that you were exposed to.
- How did these methods help you learn? Did you then learn further by yourself – how?
- How do you know you have acquired the skill?

An outline answer is provided at the end of the chapter.

Having thought about planning teaching for individual patients in some detail, we now come to some specific ideas for teaching before going on to evaluating patient teaching.

Teaching children

Teaching children requires a more detailed knowledge of how children learn at different stages of development. Theorists present various ideas of these stages and differ as to when they occur, but if you have a general idea and then acknowledge that children develop at different rates, you should be able to adapt your teaching accordingly. The important things to remember are that children do not learn in the same way as adults, and that they progress through stages of developing capability to learn.

Concept summary: Piaget's stages of cognitive development

Sensorimotor stage, ages 0 to 2

- Children are extremely egocentric (concerned only with themselves), so may not be interested in watching you.
- Children think that whatever happens is not caused by what they did, so you can't expect them to repeat a skill.
- Children have a limited concept of time, so 'in a minute' means nothing.
- At first it's out of sight, out of mind; then, later, objects have permanence, so peek-a-boo games work well, but a child still won't find his or her cup to drink out of.
- Teach through doing things *with* children and *for* them. Don't expect initiation of actions you are trying to show them.

Pre-operational stage, ages 2 to 7

- Some egocentricity remains; children think everyone experiences things the same as they do.
- Children have difficulty understanding others' points of view.
- Children tend to think they caused events and are to blame in that case.

(Continued)

(Continued)

- Animism exists – toys and teddy bears, etc. have feelings and can be hurt, so make-believe play works well.
- Group learning is limited, so you need persuasion to get children to listen to others.
- There is a lack of conservation – this means they can't focus on size, length and number, etc. together, so they see a drink in a tall thin glass as being more than the same volume in a short, wide glass.
- Teach through repetition of songs, rhymes and actions, as teaching using explanations of consequences does not work.
- Use teddies and dolls to show actions. Animals as patients in stories can be effective.
- Use actual, real equipment to demonstrate procedures. Using different 'play' items may confuse if they are different shapes (but realistic models would be useful).
- Learning through trial and error is important; children are manipulating things themselves and seeing the consequences.

Concrete operational stage, ages 7 to 11

- Children begin to develop logical thought.
- Learning that previously had to be demonstrably 'real' can now be predicted in their heads.
- Rules for action become very important, and could be useful, or not. Children will say 'You can't do that, it's not allowed.' Alternatively, you might want to set a rule for safety's sake.
- Children are less egocentric and start listening to and believing others.
- Conservation has been learned, so objects can exist in different forms and still have the same capacity or function. This can be helpful when equipment or medication change format.
- Teach by using puzzles and riddles, etc., which have rules.
- You can now discuss consequences of actions or inactions more effectively.
- But large, complex concepts will have to wait, for example infection and its effects.
- Children may not recognise the permanence of their conditions and ask when they will get better, even after your explanation.
- Children can be taught in groups and can learn from each other.

Formal operational stage, age 11 plus

- Children can now use rules creatively (and bend them).
- They can think abstractly and imagine outcomes – 'what if?'
- Children develop concern for moral and ideological causes. This sometimes gets in the way when whatever you are teaching goes against, for example, their newly discovered human rights agenda or decision to become a vegetarian.
- Emotional capacity to cope is still limited as children can't yet see their adult role.
- In learning their adult role, they will test the reality of your teaching.
- Teach through discussion and debate. Allow children to read for themselves and challenge you.
- Allow safely limited experimentation, for example deciding on their own choice of meal within a limited diet.
- Answer complex questions as children learn how to handle complex concepts.

Jean Piaget constructed his theories between 1920 and 1980. Some people who work with children believe his theories are good and sufficient to work with, but there are criticisms. It is true that, like many theorists, he does not have all the answers to cognitive development in children. To begin with, his critics point out that he did not consider social factors such as parenting and schooling in his descriptions of stages. Another issue to consider is his rather strict age groups. Some other theorists believe children reach these or similar stages much earlier than he describes. It is certainly true, of course, that children progress gradually through the developments at their own pace. You will recognise many of the points above in the children under your care. A good, readable source is www.simplypsychology. org/piaget.html.

Group teaching

Quite often, teaching in a small group of older teenagers or adults can be a most effective method to facilitate learning in health promotion. People can join in with the discussion, share experiences and ask questions of each other. By accepting an invitation to attend the group teaching session, patients and their relatives are making a commitment, and this may have a positive effect on learning because they feel that others are in the same situation. This sharing factor is influenced by the group dynamics and involves a high degree of interaction. Individuals in the group can start to apply knowledge, solve problems and develop positive attitudes. Small-group teaching also develops skills of listening, presenting ideas and persuading. It is important to maintain and support the group, giving encouragement and thereby creating a warm and friendly setting.

Activity 4.4   *Communication*

You are currently on practice experience in the community. A group of five women currently take medication for high blood pressure. They have individually attended appointments with the practice nurse for blood pressure monitoring and general health advice related to their blood pressure levels. There is a new approach for teaching patients at the GP practice. These women have been especially invited together to attend a group teaching session about weight loss. The practice nurse suggests that you run the new teaching session with her support.

• How do you go about this?

An outline answer is provided at the end of the chapter.

Whether teaching groups or individuals, at some stage you will be using printed information materials, usually leaflets, although information sheets and cards are commonly used for short instructions. There are many of these available from government or other national organisations and charities. You may be writing them yourself for your patient care areas.

Written information

A frequently used aid to teaching or information giving is the information sheet, or what is often called the 'patient information leaflet' (PIL) (Iddo and Prigat, 2004). Health professionals widely use these when involved in patient education or health promotion work.

Many leading medical charities in the UK provide support, information (patient information leaflets), teaching and research into the medical conditions that they represent. Having the details of such charities, being able to introduce patients to them and making use of the excellent teaching resources may be an invaluable resource for your patients. This may offer another teaching and learning opportunity. A short list of some useful national medical charities is included at the end of the chapter. There will be many others and, indeed, in addition you may also be able to find regional support for your patients on a local basis.

Case study: Information and support

Fred Baker is 70 years old and he has type 2 diabetes. His practice nurse found him additional information and support with the charity Diabetes UK. Fred has become a member of this charity that is involved with and campaigns on behalf of people affected by and at risk of diabetes. Fred feels cared for with this charity and has learned a great deal about his diabetes. He feels much better about managing his health and he is impressed with the research that it supports.

Recently Fred has been diagnosed with an eye condition, age-related macular degeneration (AMD). People affected suffer from loss of their central vision. While macular disease can cause serious sight loss, to other people the person affected appears completely normal. People suffering from this condition with central visual loss may still be able to see peripherally, that is seeing out of the side or corner of their eye/s. Fred is worried about how to explain this to others and that, while he likes to be independent, there are times when he may need some assistance. Once again he finds help, information and support from a charity, the Macular Society, a national charity for anyone affected by macular conditions. With the support of the helpline he finds a local macular support group, where people with AMD meet and offer information and support. Fred feels his self-esteem and understanding about this eye condition improving with help from the information leaflets/booklets that the society provides in large print.

See Chapter 5 on supporting self management.

Key issues of readability and legibility need to be considered when writing health information literature. Readability promotes meaning and understanding and depends on the choice of words and sentence length. Clarity of print and size of lettering aid the recognition and legibility of the words. The basic formula for a printed leaflet comprises: thinking of the words, deciding how many pictures and diagrams would be relevant, and selecting the size of typeface and the layout. When writing for such materials, keep to clear, simple messages (DH, 2003). Keep the intended reader focused in your mind while writing, avoid the use of jargon and define any technical words when they need to be introduced. Keep the use of abbreviations and acronyms to a minimum. Use short words and possibly consider the use of lists or bullet points to emphasise important issues. It is a good idea to pre-test the written material by giving it to someone to check that he or she can read it and understand it.

Concept summary: Written materials – top tips

- Keep simply to one subject in each leaflet.
- Keep the leaflets up to date.
- Use everyday language and explain any medical terms used.
- Write directly and inclusively – using 'you' and 'we'.
- Use present and active tenses, i.e. 'your appointment is on…' rather than 'an appointment has been made for…'.
- Write in short sentences.
- Give reasons for any instructions.
- Make the leaflets look interesting – with small blocks of text, bullet points, questions and answers – and leave some 'white' space in between writing.
- Use a plain (for example, Arial) and large enough (at least 12 or 14 point) font.
- Limit the use of bold and other decorative forms of presentation.
- Use clear illustrations rather than representational images that do not show the real thing.

More guidelines are available from DH (2003), RNIB (2004), Mencap Accessibility Team (2008) and NHS (2010).

You may also find these tips useful in deciding which leaflets to stock in the clinical area. You may notice that some are not popular with patients because they are less easy to read or perhaps contain information that is too complicated. Leaflets are freely available from charity and hospital websites and you could check out examples. The BMA (British Medical Association) gives annual awards for the best patient information leaflets (see Useful websites).

Case study: A misunderstanding

Mr Clark comes to see his practice nurse, Mo, following a visit to the dermatology clinic, having been referred there by his GP. At 85 years of age and with limited hearing, Mr Clark was pleased to report that the consultation had gone well. 'The consultant was very patient with me. He explained everything about this skin patch on my head. He told me it was a non-malignant condition and gave me a leaflet which is very helpful.'

Fortunately, Mr Clark has brought the leaflet with him and Mo reads it. It seems easy to read and quite comprehensive. However, it does say that the skin condition (basal cell carcinoma) is, in fact, malignant,

(continued)

continued . . .

albeit very slow-growing. Mo wonders whether Mr Clark has misheard, does not understand the language or is holding on to a safer diagnosis, rather than recognising that he has a cancer. In any case Mo feels that Mr Clark needs a more detailed discussion to ensure his understanding. Mo goes through the leaflet with him carefully.

Nurses teaching their patients on a one-to-one basis can make best use of leaflets by discussing them *with* the patient, pointing out the key sections that support the message they want to get across. It might be helpful to write in the margins or circle a paragraph or diagram, to reinforce or to emphasise and personalise the message as part of the discussion. Other methods of using leaflets might be to leave them clearly displayed in an open area, for example the GP practice or hospital clinic. Organising an attractive, tidy display of the leaflets is a useful technique. People can look at them and quietly select them for reading if they are too embarrassed to ask for information. They can then read through the leaflets at their own pace and, perhaps later, take any questions or points of discussion they may have to their healthcare professionals.

A benefit of written information can be that patients can refer back to the material as required. There is less of a need for patients to take notes and it can reduce anxiety levels. It can be easy and cheap to produce basic written information. Mass-produced leaflets, however, are not tailored to everyone's needs and they may contain advertising. In such instances nurses must be discerning and select appropriate leaflets for their teaching sessions. Will the leaflets be easily understood? Are they written in plain language? Are they available in other languages? Are they available in large print for visually impaired patients? Will they empower the patients? Will they encourage them to ask questions or discuss their health situations? It has to be remembered that any leaflet should be used alongside a face-to-face discussion and not used as a substitute for the health promoter.

Activity 4.5   *Communication*

You are currently on practice experience in a district general hospital in the outpatients' department. Your mentor asks if you would organise a display of PILs in one of the clinics by the end of the week. New display equipment has arrived in the department and has been unpacked ready for use. The old leaflets have been removed to a storeroom and the boxes of new leaflets are in Sister's office.

• How would you go about this?

An outline answer is provided at the end of the chapter.

Leaflets are not the only source of written material; these days more and more people are looking to the internet for health information.

Electronic media

Nurses need to be aware that many of the patients they spend time with may have accessed the internet to discover more about their health or their illness. The Office for National Statistics reported in 2015 that the internet was accessed every day or almost every day by 78 per cent of UK adults (39.3 million). Men (88 per cent) were more likely to be internet users than women (85 per cent). This compares with 35 per cent of adults in 2006 (16.2 million) when directly comparable records began. Accessing the internet using a mobile phone more than doubled between 2010 and 2012, from 24 per cent to 51 per cent and it is estimated that this will be 63 per cent of mobile phone users by 2017. This evolution in information technology is bringing huge benefits to health promotion, enabling information seeking and giving access to such information without having to contact healthcare professionals. Smartphones and tablets have become an integral part of our lives. One of the key features are health apps for smartphones and they can be helpful for improvements to health care. However, they are only as good as the information they contain. Unless the content is written by and maintained by subject experts they could be worse than useless. Not all the popular websites for health provide accurate and quality information. Any person can set up a website and some of the information given may be incorrect. It is useful for nurses to check out information on health websites to ensure that you can suggest reliable sources of information to patients. For example, if authoritative sites such as the Department of Health or the WHO give a link to other sites, they are likely to be genuine. At the Information Standard organisation, a certification scheme is available for organisations producing health and social care information that is evidence-based. Many organisations, for example NHS Choices, Patient UK or ASH, are certified by the Information Standard (www.theinformation standard.org/members). The certificate is only awarded if the information is clear, accurate, balanced, well written, accessible, evidence-based and up to date.

Hardyman et al. (2005) report that the internet on its own would be unlikely to replace person-to-person advice and support. Twenty-three per cent, almost a quarter, of the callers to a helpline for a cancer charity had already looked at the website before calling. The researchers found that the website would not totally replace the telephone helpline, that there was a need to talk to a person and that a mixture of both resources was needed (Hardyman et al., 2005).

Whichever way, and with whatever resources you decide to teach patients, you will need to measure whether the teaching has been effective.

Evaluating teaching

There are two issues in the evaluation of any teaching:

- what has been learned – the level of learning achieved;
- the quality of the teaching itself.

Learning can be evaluated through 'testing', as you know from your own learning of nursing. How you test patients may depend on their age, readiness and ability to learn as well as the content of the teaching plan. Knowledge can be tested by asking the patient to repeat the material back to you, or by giving a series of questions to answer. Some people (and often children) respond well to a quiz approach, perhaps with rewards in the form of praise or prizes. Group learning could be evaluated with a competition style of quiz, like a pub quiz. A skill can be tested by asking the patient to demonstrate it back to you.

In any situation, if a patient has not remembered accurately or fully, the teacher must accept this and give praise for trying and for what has been remembered. The material still to be learned then needs to be repeated, without blame. Positive praise enhances learning; focusing on the negative does not.

Evaluating your own teaching can be done through reflection yourself, or by asking someone else to observe you and give you feedback. In addition, ask patients to tell you what they think about your teaching. Issues to consider include:

- up-to-date material and resources;
- accuracy and whether everything important has been included;
- appropriate level (using Bloom – see page 71);
- environment conducive to learning;
- appropriate timing and speed;
- quality of written resources (see top tips, page 79);
- encouraging the patient to interact and ask questions;
- a confident manner;
- recording teaching in the patient's records.

Patient teaching is part of nursing care

It can be difficult to set aside time for teaching patients, but it is essential for patients' management of their own health (see Chapter 5). It also makes nursing care so much easier when patients are well informed.

Learning needs can be assessed and recorded at the same time as other care needs. Just asking patients why they are in the hospital, clinic or GP practice reveals a great deal about learning needs. Recording patients' own words can help nurses planning the teaching to understand what it is the patients know.

As we have discussed, making general teaching plans for groups of patients can save time in gathering information and resources. Having a good supply of written materials on display will allow patients to read first and think of questions to ask.

Making time to teach every patient needs a confident and determined approach. You could begin by thinking that every patient will need some teaching input at admission, and then at intervals until prior to discharge. This will correct a common practice of only thinking about what the patient needs to know in terms of going home. Similarly, checking on learning and teaching a little more often, each day or at each clinic or home visit perhaps, can become a part of your regular practice. Chapter 7 will explore further the relevant management elements of embedding health teaching into nursing practice.

Finally, the teaching and learning must be recorded in patients' records. You could record every teaching session or even brief opportunities to give information in your daily reporting and recording. Steven in the coronary care unit has produced a single-sheet summary of the teaching plan he devised. A copy of this sheet is amended by the nurse teaching a patient and is then inserted into the patient's notes. The nurse writes the name of the patient and the dates of teaching and signs the record.

Before we leave this chapter, we want to introduce a broader view of the patient as a member of the community as well as someone under our care. Health information is relevant to all people and, in a similar way to other skills for life such as IT skills, the skills of working with health information are increasingly useful to consumers of health.

Health literacy

The term 'health literacy' has been used in the literature for many years. Individuals with underdeveloped skills in reading and writing will not only have less exposure to traditional health education, but also less developed skills to act upon the information received. The Department of Health states that health literacy is the relationship between a person's language and numeracy levels, and her or his ability to receive, understand and process health information. Low levels of health literacy impact negatively on individuals' ability to take action to improve their health (DH, 2007). Nurses need to consider therefore that health literacy depends on the level of literacy, language and numeracy skills that their patients may have. This in turn will impact on the ability of the patients to make informed health and lifestyle choices and also to 'navigate' an increasingly complex healthcare system. The WHO points out that health literacy means much more than the ability to read a leaflet and make health appointments. It is about the cognitive and social skills involved in being a patient. The degree of health literacy will determine the ability and motivation of individuals to access and understand and use effectively the heath information in ways that will promote good health. The WHO sees health literacy as essential to empowerment (WHO, 2009). The Patient Information Forum has reported on a UK-wide survey of information providers and a group of health and education academics and practitioners have founded the Health Literacy Group. They are committed professionals who wish to raise the profile of health literacy as a remediable cause of health inequalities in England. (See Useful websites for both of these groups.)

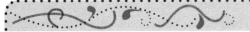

Chapter summary

This chapter has enabled you to explore and develop an understanding of some aspects of teaching patients. The chapter has focused on the organisation of teaching, which can be adapted for any care area. The ideas of readiness to learn and barriers to learning have been explored and written health materials have been examined. You need to have knowledge and comprehension of teaching and learning, follow its application to patients, analyse the component parts of the process and evaluate the importance of patient teaching to nursing care.

Activities: brief outline answers

Activity 4.1: Reflection (page 71)

You could use a method of analysis for this activity:

- list the barriers you observed;
- for each one, describe the reasons you think it occurred – how did the nurse let it happen?
- give some ideas for removing or mediating these barriers – what could the nurse have done?
- consider how you could learn from this for your future practice.

Activity 4.2: Communication (page 74)

The boy of ten with asthma is able at that age to understand, apply and even analyse information. He will be curious and questioning, perhaps showing off that he knows quite a lot already. On the negative side he may act resentfully and stubbornly refuse to cooperate. He needs to know:

- when to use the inhaler;
- how to breathe in the dose most effectively;
- what the drug does;
- how to store and clean the inhaler, and how to store the drug;
- to carry it all around safely and ready to use;
- to tell the teacher or a responsible person, such as the swimming-pool attendant, that he may need to use it.

Resources you could use include the inhaler, the drug container and the instruction leaflets that come with them, a model of the airways and a leaflet from Asthma UK.

The woman with a learning disability is less likely to learn quickly and may only achieve a lower level on Bloom's taxonomy (see page 71). She would learn better through the use of real equipment and actual demonstration than through play-acting or cartoon characters, as she does not transfer the learning very well. She needs to know:

- what the outer ear looks like;
- that earwax is normal and needed to keep the dust out;
- not to put anything into her ear;

- to wash her ears with a finger and a clean flannel;
- to tell her carer if her ears are itchy or she can't hear well;
- how to use the cream prescribed for her infection.

Resources you could use include your ear to look at, some examples of bad things to use (cotton buds, hair clips) – and let her see you throw them out, a flannel over your finger to show how she must not go deeper into the ear, and the cream so that she can see the right amount to use. Get her to use the correct method of washing.

The teenage boy's depression indicates that he is temporarily unable to learn very much, so you are going to have to instruct him with dos and don'ts rather than to try to get him to understand and analyse. He needs to know that he must:

- take the tablets at regular intervals;
- not miss any out;
- finish the course;
- not drink any alcohol until the course is finished;
- tell the doctor or nurse if he feels sick or develops a rash.

Resources you could use include the packet of tablets and the leaflet that comes with it, and a list of dos and don'ts to take away. Although he is capable of reaching higher levels on Bloom's taxonomy, his depression will blunt his ability to interact with others and to be sufficiently self-aware to cope. His parents will hopefully be involved and could set out a pattern of daily monitoring. You could encourage the parents not to do things for the boy, but to develop reminder systems such as meeting at key points in the day and using his mobile phone to send text messages.

The 82-year-old woman with diabetes seems to be a capable adult learner but may be less willing to accept yet another change to her daily life. Many elderly people would say 'I'm too old to be bothered with this.' However, she has a lack of understanding of her condition even though she has been taught previously. She may take some persuading to learn more since she thought she knew enough and now she feels overwhelmed because there is more for her to understand. She needs to know that:

- high blood sugar (when diabetes is not controlled well) means there is sugar in the tissues;
- sugar in the tissues tends to encourage bacterial growth;
- when tissue is damaged, for example blisters and cuts on the feet, infection can get in and increase;
- this means that she must look after her vulnerable feet – keep them clean and free from damage;
- she may need to consider new, better-fitting shoes;
- she needs access to a chiropodist, even just to have her toenails cut.

Resources you could use include a model or diagram of a foot showing points of potential damage, photographs of problems with feet (infections, gangrene), a leaflet from Diabetes UK and/or details of their website.

Activity 4.3: Reflection (page 75)

You may have been taught the skill by any of these methods of teaching:

- demonstration;
- supervised practice with patients;
- using models and simulated situations.

You may have learned further on your own by:

- continuing to practise handling the equipment without a patient;
- asking your mentor for opportunities to practise;
- reading more around the issue, to understand the rationale.

You will know you have acquired the skill because:

- you feel confident;
- you can do it without errors;
- you need less supervision;
- you can do it with reasonable and appropriate speed;
- you can teach it to someone else.

The same applies to the patients you teach.

Activity 4.4: Communication (page 77)

- Establish how much time there is for your teaching session. Ask if this is one of a group of sessions or the only one.
- Structure and plan the session. Balance the time between presentation of information and time for discussion. Explain your structure and schedule to the group, that is: starting at..., due to finish at ..., topics today... (make your list of the points that must be presented to remind yourself).
- Establish what the participants already understand about weight loss and find out about progress (if any) with their weight loss.
- Decide what visual aids you will use (posters? leaflets?) - are they easy to read; do they make the points that you need to present to the group? Can the women personalise this information, by making their own notes on the leaflets?
- Plan for a conclusion, which should include feedback time and questions or activities to establish what participants have learned.

Activity 4.5: Communication (page 80)

You will need to think carefully about this apparently easy activity. Maximising the effectiveness of this resource and the opportunity for the department to put across important health messages will involve some thought and planning.

- Is the new display stand in its final resting place in the clinic or do you see an alternative location? Will this new position mean better access for patients in the waiting area? Will the new proposed location meet with health and safety requirements, for example by not blocking access to fire exits?
- What are the types of clinics that run in this area of outpatients? Check out the weekly timetable for the clinics. If there are a number of different clinics running over the week you may choose to display a variety of leaflets; alternatively, you may want to propose to your mentor that the department selects a 'theme' that runs for a period of time. (There is a need to change a 'theme' regularly so that looking at the same materials doesn't become boring.) If, however, the area always has a regular clinic running in the location, for example cardiology, the selection of the patient information leaflets should be focused on linked topics.
- Plan to spend time looking through the new materials that have been ordered for the display stand; ask your mentor about this access. Look again at the 'top tips' for written materials for ideas (see page 79). You may consider carrying out a critique of the PIL materials; do you think that patients can use the materials at their own pace or with help from practitioners? You could present this critique to your mentor.

- Select from the resource box the PILs for the display stand; count them out (this keeps a crude estimate of numbers of patients acquiring the leaflets). Work out a proposed top-up system for replacing removed leaflets.

- Put the selected leaflets out before clinics start.

- Discuss with your mentor your approach to this work.

Further reading

Department of Health (2003) *Toolkit for Producing Patient Information.* London: DH. Available online at http://webarchive.nationalarchives.gov.uk/+/www.dh.gov.uk/en/Publicationsandstatistics/Publications/PublicationsPolicyAndGuidance/DH_4070141.

Although this is archived material, there is still very useful guidance to be found here.

Department of Health (2004) *Providing Patients with Better Information in Emergency Departments – Toolkit.* London: DH. Available online only at www.dh.gov.uk/en/Publicationsandstatistics/Publications/PublicationsPolicyAndGuidance/DH_4081347.

Again, this is archived material but contains useful guidance.

London, F (2012) *No Time to Teach: The Essence of Patient and Family Education for Healthcare Providers.* Online: Create Space Independent Publishing Platform.

This is an interesting American text with insight into the importance of the teaching role of the registered nurse.

Patient Education and Counseling

This is the official journal of EACH, the European Association for Communication in Healthcare, and AACH, the American Academy on Communication in Healthcare. It is an interdisciplinary international journal for patient education and health promotion researchers, managers, physicians, nurses and other healthcare providers. It has articles that are not always easy to read as the contributors write in an academic and research-based style. However, American nurse researchers lead the field in patient education, so it is worth reading to see many ideas for teaching patients, and to realise the strength of research internationally.

Protheroe, J, Nutbeam, D and Rowlands, G (2010) Health literacy: a necessity for increasing participation in health care, *British Journal of General Practice*, 59(567): 721–3.

Useful websites

http://bma.org.uk/about-the-bma/bma-library/patient-information-awards

The BMA (British Medical Association) gives annual awards for the best patient information leaflets. On this website there is a lot of information about how entries are judged.

www.healthliteracy.org.uk/why-it-is-important

This will take you to the Health Literacy Group's article, 'Why is health literacy important?'

www.pifonline.org.uk/wp-content/uploads/2013/09/PiF-Health-Literacy-Report-WEB-NEW-FINAL.pdf

The Patient Information Forum's report on a UK-wide survey of information providers.

Useful national medical charities UK:

Alzheimers Society **www.alzheimers.org.uk**

Action on Hearing Loss (RNID) **www.justgiving.com/actiononhearingloss**

Age UK **www.ageuk.org.uk**

Asthma UK **www.asthma.org.uk**

British Heart Foundation (BHF) **www.bhf.org.uk**

Diabetes UK **www.diabetes.org.uk**

Epilepsy Society **www.epilepsysociety.org.uk**

International Glaucoma Association (IGA) **www.glaucoma-association.com**

Macular Society **www.macularsociety.org**

MIND **www.mind.org.uk**

National Aids Trust **www.nat.org.uk**

National Osteoporosis Society **www.nos.org.uk**

Royal National Institute for the Blind (RNIB) **www.rnib.org.uk**

Finally, you may like to look at some of the following websites that patients can access for information. These have a range of health news, electronic leaflets and information videos on medical conditions and health problems. These websites are recommended because they give reliable health information; be cautious about using sites sponsored by health products.

www.besthealth.bmj.com

www.easyhealth.org.uk/content/about-website

www.healthtalkonline.org

www.netdoctor.co.uk

www.patient.co.uk/pils.asp

Chapter 5
Supporting self-management

continued . . . •

9. Ensures access to independent advocacy.
10. Recognises situations and acts appropriately when a person's choice may compromise their safety or the safety of others.
11. Uses strategies to manage situations where a person's wishes conflict with nursing interventions necessary for the person's safety.
14. Actively helps people to identify and use their strengths to achieve their goal and aspirations.

Chapter aims

By the end of this chapter you will be able to:

*   discuss the concept of self-management;
*   realise the personal, social and economic impact of long-term conditions on the NHS and the individual;
*   appreciate how government health policy informs the self-management of long-term conditions;
*   describe self-management models and how they support patients to self-manage their long-term conditions;
*   identify ethical issues and professional roles.

Introduction

During your practice experience you would have nursed patients suffering from **long-term conditions**. Now consider the following case study.

Case study: Increasing the level of engagement

Sophie is a 15-year-old patient who has mild learning difficulties and is suffering from epilepsy. She is frequently admitted to hospital due to poor control of her epileptic seizures. On her last admission she and her parents had a series of one-to-one consultations with the clinical nurse specialist as part of the discharge planning. The aim of the consultations was to support Sophie to develop knowledge, skills and confidence to manage her condition. During the consultations, Sophie was no longer a passive recipient of professional nursing advice as she had productive conversations with the nurse specialist in the presence of her parents on what mattered most to her. She was encouraged to actively participate in the discussions about her health, to ask questions and to air her concerns. As a result of that level of engagement, Sophie felt that she had a

continued . . .

clear and better understanding of her health condition and she no longer viewed having epilepsy as a stigma. From then on, she felt confident to take control of her own health. Sophie, in partnership with the nurse specialist and her parents, had an equal input into her personalised care plan by identifying future support needs and setting out agreed goals of care, taking into account her personal health, educational and social needs. She set out the agenda of what she was going to change to improve her health behaviour, and when and how she was going to make those changes. Together, they identified her support needs following hospital discharge. She stated that she would make full use of the internet by downloading relevant apps in order to manage her health condition more effectively. She also highlighted that following hospital discharge she would make contact with ward staff and the clinical nurse specialist either by email, telephone or text as and when she needed further advice.

This case study highlights that, by receiving active support from the clinical nurse specialist, Sophie recognised that living with epilepsy is a lifelong journey and she felt confident to self-manage her condition. She felt that receiving clear information and advice from the clinical nurse specialist helped her to develop a better understanding of the physical and emotional effects of her condition and the importance of adhering to the prescribed treatment. She felt more confident in her own ability to have a positive health impact and to improve the quality of her life. Hibbart and Gilburt (2014) support Sophie's new-found confidence. They call this process of engagement **patient activation**. They state that patients with long-term conditions who have a high level of activation are more likely to engage in positive health behaviours, and have the confidence and skills to manage their condition more effectively. Hibbart and Cunningham (2008) found that 25–40 per cent of the population with long-term conditions have low levels of activation. These patients are overwhelmed with the task of self-managing their health problems due to lack of confidence, low self-esteem (see Chapter 1: Bandura, 1977; Rotter, 1966) and a lack of problem-solving skills. These patients have experienced failures to manage their own health condition effectively and, as a result, they have developed a heavy reliance/dependancy on health professionals for the management of their health condition.

Self-management of long-term conditions is at the heart of current health policy, urging healthcare professionals to support and help people with long-term conditions to take control of those conditions. Nurses have been identified by the government as the key professionals to give such help. This chapter will outline the concept of self-management and epidemiological data for long-term conditions. It will also discuss various models of self-management and relevant health policy that nurses can use as a framework to build self-management programmes. In doing so, nurses are aiming to support patients to take responsibility for their own health by developing problem-solving and decision-making skills, the ability to work collaboratively with healthcare practitioners and the ability to set realistic daily personal plans to enhance their quality of life. The chapter will also address the ethical issues nurses have to consider when they are involved in the promotion of self-management for patients with long-term conditions.

Case study: Becoming an expert patient

Annie, who is 45 years old, describes herself as youthful looking, stylish and eloquent. She was diagnosed with Crohn's disease ten years ago. At the time, she was working as a secondary school teacher and was a single mother of two children. She and her husband had divorced the year before her diagnosis. Recently, Annie became an expert patients' educator for Crohn's disease. During one of the sessions that she delivered to a group of ten participants, all of them suffering with the same condition, Annie reminisced:

'When first I was diagnosed with Crohn's disease I had problems of accepting my diagnosis and readjusting my lifestyle. I felt very anxious and fearful about my future. I was in turmoil about whether to share my health news with my children. I was fearful of how this could affect our relationship. I kept it to myself for one year. Eventually the time came to speak to them. They both used the internet and found out everything one can about Crohn's disease. The children are a great support. However, Crohn's took over our lives.'

Annie recalls that she was losing her self-confidence and self-esteem. She started to lose control of her life and eventually she lost her job:

'I thought that I would be teaching until retirement age. In the early days I felt constantly worn out and depressed. I could not go out unless I knew that I could access toilet facilities immediately when the need arose. I used to dread when I had to visit my gastroenterology consultant. As soon as I entered the door of the consultation room I used to feel like a six-year-old going to see the head teacher. I used to feel very vulnerable and completely disempowered. He had complete control over the management of my condition. He was making all the decisions based on the medical presentation and his professional expertise. For example, on each visit he would always ascertain how often I opened my bowels daily and then he would proceed to readjust my medication. At the time I felt that my consultant did not value my personal experience and the expertise I had developed over time about Crohn's disease. My dream was that one day I would walk into the consultation room and be able to deal with the situation better. I wanted to be heard and to participate in the decision-making process about my own health. I wanted to be acknowledged as myself and not as the person with Crohn's.'

Self-management

During your clinical experience you may have seen cases similar to Annie's. This case study clearly illustrates that Annie, in the early days of her journey with Crohn's, did not have any control over the management of her condition. It also highlights her desire to be an active participant in the decision-making process. She explicitly wanted to be in charge of her life and own health. The case study raises many pertinent issues (lack of control and confidence, vulnerability, non-participation in decision making and unequal power between professionals and patients), which have a huge impact on the life and health outcomes of individuals who suffer from long-term conditions. Annie wanted the medical and allied health care professionals to recognise that she had insightful expertise of her own condition based on her personal experience of living with Crohn's disease. The *Five Year Forward View* (NHS England, 2014) recognises that patients are experts in their own long-term condition and play a vital role in the management of their own health. Long-term conditions are a central task of the NHS and it has set out the future vision for their management. It strongly advocates patient empowerment and equal input between professionals and patients to plan, implement and review care, rather than the traditional provision of sporadic and unconnected episodes of care.

In your career so far you may have observed that, while drugs are necessary in the management of illness, they offer only partial solutions to the problem and to the medical management of chronic conditions. Annie clearly wanted to take back some control over her life. She did not want Crohn's disease to dominate her life and the life of her children. She wanted to gain her own personal identity and dignity.

The case study illustrates succinctly the medicalisation of health in the early years of Annie's condition. She was seen as the patient with Crohn's rather than as the person with life experience, personal achievement and accomplishments. The focus was on controlling the disease rather than on the promotion of good health and well-being as advocated by the NMC. The doctor was in charge and the patient was a passive, docile and obedient participant. However, current clinical practice is changing under the influence of evolved cultural and professional values and government policy. The Department of Health aims to improve the health of people who suffer from long-term diseases by urging local community health organisations to empower patients by implementing health promotion strategies that encourage self-management. NHS England (2016) identifies a tripartite partnership between NHS England, clinical commissioning groups and local authorities to provide comprehensive and high-quality care for people with long-term conditions.

Self-management, as a concept, is geared towards people of all ages (children, adolescents, adults and older people) who are suffering from long-term conditions, for example diabetes, arthritis, asthma, depression, schizophrenia, cerebral palsy and epilepsy, as well as towards their carers and families. It aims to increase patients' independence by improving their quality of life. It also aims to enable them to be active and productive citizens by taking control of their own health and personal lives.

This means that you, as a nurse, should undertake health promotion interventions (see the section 'Models of self-management' later in this chapter) that enable patients with long-term health conditions to maximise their health potential and quality of life rather than just to control and manage their illnesses. Patients have to develop self-reliance mechanisms by being proactive rather than passive recipients of healthcare. They have to find solutions to everyday problems and not submit to lives that are dominated by their disease. As a nurse in partnership with other professionals, you are a key player in facilitating this transition.

Epidemiological evidence supporting self-management

As a student nurse, independent of your field of practice, you will have nursed patients who suffered from a variety of long-term conditions under the supervision of your mentor.

- Note down some of the conditions you have come across during your clinical experience.
- Consider what many of these patients have in common.

An outline answer is provided at the end of the chapter.

In the UK, and globally, life expectancy improved steadily over the twentieth century and continues to do so. It is estimated that women born in the UK between 2004 and 2006 will live on average to 81 years of age, while men will reach the age of 77 years.

Living longer is good news. However, as we live longer, the chances of developing diseases that will have a long-term effect on our health, such as arthritis, heart conditions, diabetes, dementia and respiratory problems, to mention just a few, are increasing for both sexes. These conditions are a threat to health status and cause impairment to the quality of life due to disability.

It is estimated that today in the UK an alarming 17.5 million adults are living with a long-term condition (DH, 2004b) and approximately 30 per cent of these patients also have a mental health problem (Naylor et al., 2012). The Department of Health estimates that 45 per cent of those who suffer from long-term conditions will suffer from more than one condition, for example a person with diabetes may also have circulatory and ophthalmic problems. This increased prevalence of long-term conditions results in:

- an increased number of hospital admissions and long hospitalisation, accounting for 70 per cent of hospital bed occupancy;
- an increased number of consultations with GPs, being responsible for 50 per cent of all GP consultations;
- the overall NHS expenditure in England on the care and treatment of long-term conditions accounting for 70 per cent of the total allocated NHS budget;
- people with long-term conditions having increased levels of absenteeism from work;
- long-term conditions being more prevalent among the lower socio-economic groups (lower income).

These national statistics are supported by the WHO, which forecasts that, if long-term diseases are not successfully managed by 2020, they will be the most expensive problem for healthcare systems across the world. Long-term health problems are costly in terms of both the medical care needed and the loss of national productivity because of time off work. A long-term condition is also a great burden to the individual as it causes both physical suffering and social disadvantage.

The WHO (2013) set an objective to reduce mortality from four major preventable diseases, namely cancer, cardiovascular disease, diabetes and chronic lung disease, by 25 per cent by the year 2025, using the statistics from the year 2010 as a baseline. This is known as the '25 by 25 goal'. To achieve this objective, the WHO has identified the following areas as designated targets for improvement: hypertension, obesity, diabetes, tobacco smoking, salt and sodium intake, physical inactivity and harmful levels of alcohol intake. The WHO requires all countries to develop and implement policies to meet this objective and to set their own targets. The UK government has agreed to implement the WHO's objective and targets in this regard. The 25 per cent reduction, which could be easily achieved in the developed world, may be difficult to achieve in the developing world because of the diverse economic situations and the healthcare infrastructure/ provision of the different countries. A report on the global progress of this initiative affirms this variation. It notes that, while some countries are on target to achieve the goal, others are still far from meeting the global targets (WHO, 2014). However, it could arguably be seen as a not very ambitious target for the United Kingdom, as a country that ranks as the fifth wealthiest country globally with an advanced healthcare system and health promotion provision. The PROMISE research study undertaken by the Richmond Group of Charities (2016), which is based on the WHO's set target '25 by 25', found that, in the UK, this target is achievable among women but only 22 per cent among men. This difference could be attributed to men and women's different attitudes towards health. For example, typically, women will seek medical advice and support earlier than men.

As a practitioner at the front line of healthcare provision, you will have to tackle these problems by being the steering force for implementing self-management initiatives at the grass roots of clinical practice. You therefore need to reorientate your clinical practice from 'disease management' to a 'health-enhancing' approach.

You need to act as a facilitator, which means that you have to develop new skills and to adopt a new culture of practice with the appropriate attitudes and behaviours to support patients to be independent and self-caring (see Chapters 7 and 8).

Health policy context of self-management for chronic conditions

Current government policy provides nurses with a framework and guidance on how to accomplish this transformation of practice. The government document *High Quality Care for All: The Next Stage Review Final Report* (DH, 2008b) sets out the agenda for self-management. It states that the NHS has to focus not only on the treatment of disease but also on health improvement. The subsequent two documents, *Your Health, Your Way: A Guide to Long-term Conditions and Self-care* (DH, 2009) and *Improving the Health and Wellbeing of People with Long-term Conditions* (DH, 2010a), provide further evidence for the implementation of a self-management approach by healthcare professionals.

These policies aim to produce better health outcomes and improve the quality of life for people with long-term conditions, slow the progression of their conditions and reduce disability by empowering and supporting them to understand their conditions, to determine their own health needs and to be able to make informed choices about their health.

The policies have to be applauded for steering health professionals towards a health-promoting practice. However, their implementation at a national and local level is fragmented and focused on the medical model of health (see Chapter 1), rather than on a holistic and wellness model of health. There is a need for health professionals to embrace the concept of self-management by endorsing the Ottawa Charter principles (WHO, 1986) as discussed in Chapter 1 (see pages 14–15).

Policies on their own are not sufficient to improve the health of people living with long-term conditions. There is a need to reform and reorientate the current provision of health and social care to meet the health needs and expectations of the individual and the population as a whole. The UK NHS, along with other global health systems, such as those in the USA and countries within the European Union, is slow to adapt to society's cultural diversity (see Chapter 7) and changing health needs. The traditional NHS system is fragmented and services are struggling to keep pace with current demographic pressures. During your practice experience you may already have witnessed the poor coordination of services between GPs, hospital-based specialists, hospital and community across all fields of practice. This division compromises integration of care. Nurses must actively lobby government for delivery of an innovative, preventative and responsive seamless service, which is a fundamental requirement for people suffering from long-term conditions. There is a strong need for active integration of health promotion into the care pathways as well as for the public, private and voluntary sectors to work together to support people with long-term conditions to make informed choices and take decisions that improve their health and well-being. There is an urgent case, and need, under the current economic climate of financial austerity, for a robust approach to plan and **commission** economically viable and **sustainable** health services at a national and local level, by setting clear and measurable objectives for health promotion programmes and by adopting stringent methods to evaluate the quality and impact of health promotion on health improvement for people with long-term conditions. The then coalition government's reform of health and social care provision in England, which was launched on 1 April 2013, places long-term conditions under the responsibility of NHS England, which has to produce plans and policies outlining what it will do to support self-management for people with long-term conditions to achieve better health (DH, 2012a). Northern Ireland, Scotland and Wales have made similar arrangements to meet the health needs of their own populations (see Chapter 6). A document from the Self Care Forum (2013) advocates for a 'whole systems' approach across the NHS to empower patients to self-care in a supportive environment. The mandate envisages that adopting a cohesive self-care strategy will safeguard the existence of the NHS, not only for the present generation of people but also for future generations. To enable this to materialise in practice a six-point blueprint has been developed.

- *Recognise that supporting self care can create capacity in general practice for longer consultations.*
- *For all healthcare professionals to support self care behaviour at every contact.*

- *Adopt a self care aware conversation in all consultations.*
- *Implement the NHS Constitution at practice level to underpin support for self care.*
- *Support Patient Participation Groups to implement the National Association of Patient Participation programme supporting self care for the practice population.*
- *Encourage healthcare professionals to enable patients to self care by developing national and local incentive schemes.*

(Self Care Forum, 2013)

The six-point blueprint encourages interprofessional working and the development of close partnerships between patients, families and professionals. It also stipulates that health professionals, by recognising the potential long-term benefits of self-care to the patient and to the NHS, have to re-evaluate and remodel their daily professional practice in order to facilitate capacity for supporting self-care. However, the implementation of the six-point blueprint as a model to support self-management for long-term conditions requires a strong organisational commitment to self-care, funding for longer consultations, and resources for professional development to enable staff to engage in meaningful health conversations to support self-care behaviour. Nurses, as providers of 24-hour care and as patients' **advocates**, must embrace this opportunity to take a leadership role in the development of national and local schemes to support self-management. Patients need also to have educational opportunities to develop assertive skills and to be confident to negotiate care with health professionals.

The Department of Health identifies nurses as the key professionals responsible for providing health promotion interventions to enable patients to self-manage the complexities of their conditions. The above-mentioned health strategies in conjunction with NICE guidelines and national service frameworks (NSFs) (diabetes, cancer, mental health, long-term conditions) provide nurses with a framework that informs and shapes the development of a 'self-management practice'.

Underpinning principles of supporting self-management for long-term conditions

Activity 5.2   *Reflection and critical thinking*

Reflect on three patients with three different chronic conditions whom you have nursed during your practice experience, for example, patients suffering from arthritis, diabetes and Parkinson's disease. Now consider the therapeutic conversations you have had with them and their families. What were their expressed views?

- Were they happy to be in hospital?
- What health information did they receive and from whom?

(continued)

continued . . .

- Were they satisfied with the health information they received?
- Did they feel that NHS provision at the local level met their needs?
- Did they receive any professional support when they were discharged home?
- How did the professionals who cared for them encourage self-management?

An outline answer is provided at the end of the chapter.

Reflecting on the activity, you may conclude that the conversations revealed the following common themes.

- *Patients taking responsibility for their own health management: how can you facilitate this?* You need to ensure that patients have the ability to seek, understand and evaluate the necessary health information to manage their personal health. Therefore, you must ensure that you are familiar with national and local resources and how you provide that information to patients (see Chapter 4). Is the state discharging responsibility to the individual? Consider the ethical and legal issues. Do the health system and the current political ideologies promote patients' rights? Can patients identify local resources and make choices about their health? Can they recognise personal limitations or needs for support? This is very relevant when you are nursing patients with mental health problems and learning disabilities, or adolescents whose health and well-being have been compromised by long-term conditions. Are they able to exercise their autonomy? Do they have the mental capacity to make informed decisions? In partnership with other health professionals you always have to establish mental capacity. It is important to engage patients and families in the management of their health. You should also ensure that there are policies in place to safeguard patients' privacy and confidentiality – for example, when accessing **telehealth** is their confidentiality safeguarded? You should always act as patients' advocate.

- *Patients feeling confident in their own ability to take control of their own health: how can you promote self-efficacy?* (See Chapter 1.) Do you need to address health inequalities? Have patients the ability and knowledge to set realistic goals and priorities and to solve health problems? Can they be trusted to do the right thing? What is your role and the role of the other health professionals (see Chapter 1)? The voluntary and community sectors play an important role in increasing people's independence by providing advice and information about equipment and tools for self-management – for example, the provision of self-monitoring devices for blood glucose levels. Do you know how patients might gain access to such equipment?

- *Providing patients with information and education on risks and strategies to improve their health in and of itself is not sufficient.* For example, living with a long-term condition is emotionally challenging (often engendering feelings of frustration, anger or depression). Therefore, in collaboration with other professionals, you need to consider how to sustain motivation and confidence by, for example, referring patients to assertiveness or counselling courses. Motivational interviewing, as one example, is a client-centred counselling technique that enables patients to overcome their ambivalence about changing behaviour and supports self-efficacy (Rollnick et al., 2008). Many patients may also feel segregated and socially isolated due to their conditions. In such cases you need to promote integration by referring patients to self-help local groups and to encourage involvement in **community development** initiatives or projects.

- *Nurses must respect and value patients' personal experience and knowledge of their own illnesses.* Now consider whether lay knowledge can have equal credibility and validity to professional expert knowledge. Nurses must support patients to develop a positive self-image and enable them to become more autonomous in the management of their own health. Finding out patients' individual strengths and listening to their personal experience is very important as this will give you the platform from which to build on their existing knowledge to further support self-management. Do patients have the ability to communicate effectively with professionals? Are they in a position to negotiate culturally sensitive services that meet their health needs? You need to reflect on the socialisation of nursing culture and to evaluate evidence of patients' participation and engagement in the decision-making process. Do you know what courses are available in your locality to guide patients to increase their confidence in self-management? For example, patients may benefit from developing health literacy skills and computer skills.

These themes highlight the complexity of self-management and the diversity of skills and activities required for successful self-management. They also indicate that nurses need to clarify their professional accountability and redefine the nursing role because self-management involves collective action, promotes individual choice and equalises the power between professionals and patients.

In summary, good self-management is underpinned by the following principles.

- Knowledge about the condition and monitoring its progression.

- Active participation in the decision-making process and negotiation in planning, implementing and evaluating self-management.

- Working in partnership with healthcare professionals and significant others, for example carers, to make decisions regarding health outcomes.

- Confidence to manage their physical, emotional and social lives and to access/use support services.

- Adopting healthy lifestyles and healthy behaviours.

These principles indicate that there is a need for you as a nurse to rethink and re-evaluate your daily nursing practice.

A practice that promotes self-management for long-term conditions requires that you establish ongoing, good-quality, interactive relationships with your patients and their families and carers, which are built on mutual respect and trust. Provide them with the opportunity to discuss anxieties, worries and concerns with you. However, do not assume that lay people believe that professionals know best. Patients sometimes receive conflicting and contradictory advice from professionals, such as on the issue of dairy foods affecting Crohn's disease. You must develop an evidence-based practice.

Develop a personalised self-management plan (see Chapter 7). Patients are entering into an equal partnership with healthcare professionals. Health outcomes and realistic goals are set by negotiation and mutual agreement. Progress is reviewed constantly by both parties. You need to ensure that agreement is reached by patients exercising autonomy, freedom of choice and voluntary consent.

Make sure that you deliver patient-centred education. Educational activities should be sensitive to cultural diversity and individual values and beliefs. You have to be prepared to encounter negative feelings from some patients who may resent and reject your health advice on the basis that they are 'being told what to do'. They may feel frustrated and find it difficult to conform and change their behaviour due to socio-economic factors such as lack of money or job opportunities. This highlights the importance of devising a truly personalised education that is tailor-made to patients' individual life circumstances and personal attributes, and builds on their strengths and weakness.

Gain active patient participation in the decision-making process by building patients' confidence and self-esteem and sustaining motivation. Ensure that every patient feels confident and competent to put the advice into practice by the development of skills, such as a diabetic patient becoming able to readjust his or her insulin dosage when meeting friends socially over drinks. However, you need to consider whether patients have the cognitive and emotional skills to make informed decisions. You need to question what opportunities patients have to influence care policy and guidelines. It may be said by professionals that they welcome patients' views, but much consultation is really only placatory.

Enable patients to take responsibility and control of their own health by developing problem-solving skills. You should not assume that all patients want to be responsible for their health at all times. Due to changes in personal circumstances following a 'flare-up' of their condition, a patient will feel very ill, vulnerable and unable to cope. He or she may feel despondent and disheartened and may rely on the professionals to make decisions on his or her behalf. Development of coping skills is at the heart of self-management as you are aiming to transform your patient from a sufferer to a manager.

Nurses involved in supporting patients to self-manage their long-term conditions must consider these ways of working. Patients' autonomy, freedom of choice, voluntarism, participation in decision making, responsibility and the ability to take control of their own health are the essence of health promotion practice. Patients, their families and significant others are viewed as your equal partners.

Models of self-management education

When supporting patients to self-manage their condition, how do you structure and shape your health promotion practice? As seen earlier, health policy will be instrumental in guiding your practice. Additionally, nurses, in collaboration with other health professionals, can facilitate the process of self-management by adopting the following models:

- Expert Patients Programme;

- structured education programmes (for example, for diabetes);

- empowerment.

All of these models incorporate many common activities based on health promotion theory (see Chapter 1), which aim to support and help patients to take control of their conditions and to promote good health.

In the UK, these models have informed the design of many self-management programmes, such as those for diabetes, substance and alcohol misuse, and pain.

Have you noticed that self-management is a tertiary level prevention, as identified by Tannahill (1985) (see Chapter 1)? The patients already have the disease and you aim to support and facilitate them to cope with their disease and to improve their quality of life. However, as a nurse, you have to remember that not all patients with long-term conditions will have the same level of health needs (see Chapter 7).

Even though all models have the same core aim(s) and they utilise similar health promotion theory, they differ in terms of who is involved in their delivery.

Expert Patients Programme

Case study: Expert Patients Programme (EPP)

Mick is a 67-year-old man who has suffered from arthritis for the past 35 years. He is a retired self-employed gas central heating engineer. He has been married to Monica for 45 years and has two sons and two grandsons. Mick's main hobbies are sailing and ballroom dancing.

Despite suffering pain and experiencing various degrees of stiffness and difficulty in using his hands, he worked until retirement age. He has been able to adapt and manage his arthritis with the support of his wife, consultant, physiotherapist, GP and practice nurse.

During a routine consultation with the practice nurse he was told about the Expert Patients Programme. He recalls:

'I got very excited as I felt that I had all the qualifications to be a peer educationalist. I like talking to and interacting with people of all cultures through my work and, not to forget, I've suffered from arthritis for 35 years.

I registered to attend a local course run by my PCT in a church hall near the town centre. I enjoyed the course and I found it fascinating. I learned a lot and I found that the participants had many things in common. Things such as taking painkillers before exercise activity, writing down questions to ask during GP visits and remembering to take prescriptions on holiday.'

(continued)

continued . . .

Mick attended the EPP course and he is now a voluntary peer educator, helping to run other courses. He evaluated the course as follows:

'The EPP gave me the licence to make informed decisions for myself. It built up my in-depth knowledge and understanding about my medication and potential complications of my condition. The course had a generic approach to fit with everybody's needs. One has to appreciate that the participants are at different stages with their condition. I learned how important it is to accept my condition (as there is no other alternative). Now I have learned to ventilate my feelings. I used to get on with things until I couldn't cope, while now I find it easy to express my own feelings to others. I no longer feel isolated.'

He enjoys being a volunteer peer educator:

'As a peer educator I feel that I can share my personal experience and learning with others. This is important as a lot of the things we (patients) experience are common to us all, even though we may suffer with different conditions. I am able to support and help other people. When a participant has a problem we discuss this as a group and all of us make suggestions how to deal with it.

Each week we set achievable, realistic goals for participants. The course allows people to have realistic expectations from themselves, for example you can exercise by taking the grandchildren for a walk in the park instead of expecting to run a marathon! It encourages participants to do something for themselves rather than expect professionals or the system to do it for them.

EPP can be a social event and it helps you to have a laugh without undermining the seriousness of the course.'

The case study gives a succinct account of the EPP concept and highlights how it supports patients to self-manage their long-term conditions. It is important to realise that the EPP is taught by lay people who have long-term conditions themselves: peer education is a key part of the model. People are given training to enable them to teach groups and there is a system of support for them to perform this role.

The EPP is a government initiative that has the support and recognition of the WHO. Since 2002, following the recommendations of the Wanless report (2002), it is delivered as a free programme by the NHS for people who suffer with long-term conditions. However, its origins can be traced back to the 1990s, when the voluntary sector introduced the notion of lay-led self-management for chronic conditions. Currently, EPP courses are provided by over half of local community health organisations in England. The EPP is also provided by all local health boards in Wales and is part of the health policy for Scotland.

The Arthritis Self-Management Programme is considered to be the prototype of the EPP self-management course, dating back to 1979. It is a community-based programme for people who suffer with rheumatoid arthritis, osteoarthritis, lupus and fibromyalgia. The programme has been evaluated over the years using randomised trials. The evaluation results indicate that participants reduced their pain, and sometimes their disability, reduced the uptake of NHS services and, overall, improved their quality of life (Lorig et al., 1993).

The Substance and Alcohol Misuse (SAM) course, used in the field of mental health, is another example of an EPP programme. It offers people who are recovering from drug and alcohol misuse the opportunity to learn skills that enable them to integrate successfully back into the community. This is achieved by raising participants' self-confidence and morale, and sustaining their motivation to change. The course teaches them a variety of techniques that enable them to organise their day-to-day activities constructively by setting realistic goals and making action plans. It provides participants with valuable tools and techniques that enable them to improve communication with their families, friends and healthcare professionals, and to gain the necessary skills to seek paid or voluntary employment or to pursue further education.

There are EPP programmes for general groups of patients, for those with conditions such as pain, and for carers. They are offered in modified forms to meet the needs of young people and people with learning difficulties.

Evaluation of the EPP is positive. It indicates that participants can improve their quality of life and minimise deterioration of their conditions. They are able to adopt healthy lifestyles (better diet and increased physical activity), to try new things and make important life-changing decisions because the course has increased their self-awareness and self-worth. However, evaluation has also indicated some shortcomings. Making the programme available to patients is seen as being labour-intensive and time-consuming by local NHS organisations. The EPP is helpful for some individuals and is valued as one of the options for long-term conditions. However, the course content does not acknowledge the broader social issues and needs that are relevant to people living with long-term conditions. For example, it does not address welfare issues and how to negotiate benefits relevant to people who are unable to work or who may need assistance to return to work. There is a need for a collaborative action between NHS, Social Services and the Department for Works and Pensions to address these issues that are pertinent to many patients with long-term conditions. The programme tends to attract patients who are well-educated, white and middle class, leading to a failure to address the wider socio-economic issues and complexities of living with long-term conditions and therefore, arguably, increasing inequalities. The inclusion of the 'living wills' as part of the course content has also raised concerns by some participants as some aspects are considered to be emotive and inappropriate (National Primary Care Research and Development Centre, 2007). There is also concern in relation to clinical management of diseases; for example, patients with diabetes have not always been able to control effectively their diabetes or their diet. This highlights the need for patient education programmes led by professional experts (Cabe et al., 2006).

Structured education programmes

Structured education programmes are set up by care services for patients with certain conditions and are offered to patients and carers. They are run by healthcare professionals who have professional expertise and experience pertinent to the long-term condition in question.

The educators are mainly nurse specialists, practice nurses, physiotherapists and dieticians. However, other healthcare professionals may be involved, depending on the nature of the condition, such as podiatrists, pharmacists, occupational therapists and doctors.

Examples of structured education programmes include:

- DAFNE (Dose Adjustment for Normal Eating) – for those with insulin-dependent diabetes;
- DESMOND (Diabetes Education and Self Management for Ongoing and Newly Diagnosed) – for those with non-insulin-dependent diabetes;
- X-PERT – for those with diabetes (not the same as the EPP);
- Challenging Your Condition – for those with arthritis.

Others are set up when health professionals consider there is a need. The names of some programmes are often made up locally; even the diabetes programmes may be redesigned for local use and given a local name, such as BERTIE in Bournemouth and WINDFAL at the Whittington hospital, London.

The programmes are structured to support patients in self-managing their conditions. Their curricula are provided by professionals and designed to meet the standards of self-management as outlined in the policies discussed previously. This ensures uniformity of all programmes irrespective of where they are delivered as they meet and fulfil national standards. This also enhances participants' confidence that they are attending approved, worthwhile programmes.

It is estimated that these programmes are the preferred choice of the majority of healthcare organisations throughout the UK in their effort to promote self-management among patients suffering from long-term conditions. They are delivered predominantly in local community health organisations, for example a community health centre, although some are offered in hospitals by their specialist teams. Nurses caring for patients need to be aware of the availability of relevant local programmes, their start dates and venues, in order to arrange for patients to attend.

Typically, the programmes run over a number of weeks (often six weeks) and each session is of two to three hours' duration. The sessions are interactive and each group consists of approximately ten participants.

The curricula usually address three areas:

- medical management of the condition – for example, participants will be educated on how to manage their medication and how to monitor their peak flow or blood glucose levels;
- role management – for example, delegation of responsibility to others, such as asking a partner to do the weekly shopping;
- emotional management – coping with anger, fatigue.

Inherent to the education programme is the development of problem-solving skills, decision making, resource utilisation, forming a partnership with the health professionals and taking actions in reasonable steps (action planning). This can be illustrated by the following case study.

Case study: A structured education model

Olu is a 56-year-old man of African origin who was diagnosed with bipolar depression at the age of 25 and for the past two years has suffered with hypertension. He is employed and often works up to 50 hours per week. Because of work pressures, he eats a lot of fast food for convenience. He cannot reduce his weight as he does not have time to exercise. Since his diagnosis two years ago, he is worried that he may die of a heart attack. He takes his own blood pressure readings but, because of work commitments, he finds it difficult to visit his GP. Recently his blood pressure readings were constantly elevated and he became very agitated. His wife became very concerned and texted Olu's community psychiatric nurse, who made a domiciliary visit to review Olu's mental health. During consultation it was established that Olu self-manages 'his bipolar' quite well. However, his blood pressure and related lifestyle were the main issues.

The community psychiatric nurse advised Olu and his wife to make an appointment to see the GP. Following this consultation his wife made an appointment for him to see his GP the following day. During the consultation he was advised to see the practice nurse with a view to enrolling on the structured patient education programme run by the practice nurse for hypertensive patients. Olu was seen by the practice nurse and arrangements were made to attend the course. She also communicated with Olu's community psychiatric nurse, informing him of the agreed plan of action. After completion of the course Olu's mental and physical health improved as he was able to self-manage his hypertension by the development of the following skills.

- ***Problem solving****: he is able to follow and adhere to a care plan agreed between himself and his GP, practice nurse, pharmacist and dietician. He now checks and records his blood pressure readings regularly. He also takes a small cooler bag to work that he packs with his lunch.*

- ***Decision making****: he has negotiated with his employer to be transferred to another department within the company and has reduced his working hours. He has set realistic exercise goals to fit with his daily life.*

- ***Using resources****: Olu uses the internet to update his knowledge about hypertension. He now visits his local library and is using the library's databases for research articles.*

- ***Partnership with the health professionals****: during visits to the GP and practice nurse he always uses his health diary (blood pressure recordings, medication regime and nutrition intake) to discuss his progress. He and his wife now write down a list of questions to ask the healthcare professionals.*

- ***Action planning****: Olu ensures that he stays healthy by adopting a healthy lifestyle and reducing his stress levels by taking time out to relax. He has set goals to improve his eating and exercise behaviour, and he has a weekly plan. He now emails his community psychiatric nurse regularly and, at his own suggestion, has joined the local over-50s' group for park walks. He and his wife have taken up a new hobby, growing their own vegetables in an allotment rented from the local authority. Both are members of the community's allotment club and they are now active members of the community.*

The structured education model allows health professionals to design a curriculum for gaining knowledge and skills, and developing attitudes enabling self-management. Nurses quite often meet patients who need a bit of a push to start helping themselves with their ongoing health conditions. Some rely too much on the actions of professionals to help them, and are perhaps afraid to take charge of their lives. Patients may be reluctant to change. Such programmes increase patients' quality of life and functionality, their adherence to their treatment, their self-care plan and they make good use of health services. However, employers have to provide educational opportunities and support to health professionals to develop their role as teachers and health educators. Nurses need support from management to create working opportunities (beyond their daily clinical workload) and they need time for them to undertake such a role.

Empowerment

The EPP and structured education programmes empower patients and their families to take control of their long-term condition as a core aim. Empowerment is the hub of health promotion and over the last 20 years it has been seen as one of the most significant innovations in the management of long-term conditions. An empowerment approach strengthens patients' abilities to pursue effective self-management programmes. We will consider the theory supporting empowerment.

Case study: Empowerment

Robert is a 19-year-old university student who studies engineering. He shares a flat with his girlfriend Mary near the university and both enjoy a very active social life. Robert is a keen rugby player and enjoys a variety of sports. Prior to his university course he lived with his parents and two younger siblings. At 12 years old he was diagnosed with type 1 diabetes (insulin-dependent). As part of the initiative for involving service users in his university's health faculty, he has been invited to speak to a group of student nurses about his health journey of living with diabetes as a child and an adolescent, and his progress from being a passive patient to becoming an empowered patient.

Robert tells the students:

'When first diagnosed with insulin-dependent diabetes I found it very difficult to cope with the challenges of living with diabetes. As a 12-year-old I felt very frightened, frustrated and angry. I found it difficult to discuss this with my parents, who became very overprotective, or with my siblings, who felt that I was receiving special parental attention and favouritism, and this caused a strain on our relationships. Due to my diabetes I was teased by my peers at school. I started to blame myself for my personal failing and I felt isolated.

On reflection, my initial experience of managing my diabetes was overall very mechanistic and prescriptive in nature. I was following a management regime that was determined and prescribed by my consultant and his team and my mother. The health information and written materials I received were impersonal, generic and didactic. I had no autonomy. I had to adapt my lifestyle to fit my diabetic care as recommended by the healthcare professionals

continued . . .

(consultant, nurse, dietician) and my parents, especially my mother. I lost my independence and freedom to enjoy my childhood. At the age of 14 I had problems with self-image and felt stigmatised by my peers. I started to rebel by not taking my insulin! I wanted to be normal and conformed to peer pressure by experimenting with cigarette smoking and alcohol intake, resulting in family disputes and frequent hospital admissions. My school attendance was problematic due to my frequent hospitalisation. During hospital appointments the health professionals were mainly interacting with my parents and I was almost invisible until the day when, during a doctor's consultation, my mother and I started to argue over my insulin therapy. The consultant asked to see me on my own. I was able to ventilate my feelings and express my thoughts. He showed empathy and respect, and treated me as an autonomous person who can make rational decisions and is able to take responsibility for my own health. The fact that the doctor listened and took notice of me gave me confidence and finally I had a voice. I was an active participant in the decision-making process, working in partnership with my parents and health professionals. I was assigned to a diabetes specialist nurse whom I was able to phone for advice and with whom I developed a good professional relationship. Receiving that support enabled me to take charge of my health, focus on my education, enjoy life and not carry the label of diabetes around with me. I was a normal person accepting my condition. My diabetes did not dictate who I was – it simply became part of my day-to-day living. Today, in contrast, my diabetes management gives me flexibility and I can be spontaneous in my daily activities without having to think constantly about my diabetes. I feel confident and in control. I met my girlfriend, Mary, when we were 16 and she plays an active and supportive role. This change took place as both of us participated in a number of patient education programmes, which are widely available, easily accessible, informative and non-threatening. They emphasise the role of the patient in the decision-making process and they validate our own experience and knowledge of diabetes.

Another significant change that has empowered me is the advent of a collaborative team approach to care. The healthcare team offers a wide spectrum of interprofessional expertise and experience. Nowadays, I am able to devise management plans that I can adapt to my own personal lifestyle, needs, wants and desires without compromising the fundamental medical treatment required for my diabetes.'

Robert's case study reiterates that empowerment is at the hub of self-management and demonstrates how empowered patients can control their long-term conditions and can lead a fulfilled life.

Tones and Tilford (2001) provide nurses and other health professionals with an empowerment model known as Tones' empowerment model. The model is widely used in the promotion of self-management. It illustrates that health education leads to empowerment and is based on the notion that the acquisition of health knowledge and skills that are sensitive to the individual's culture, values and beliefs can raise an individual's **critical consciousness**. This is a term first used by the Brazilian educationalist Paulo Freire; critical consciousness is the level at which individuals are able to view objectively the reality of their health status. They have the confidence, self-esteem and self-efficacy to challenge the politics of health and achieve political change, leading to equitable and holistic health. In the case of self-management, a knowledgeable patient can influence health policy at the local and national levels. Robert is able to debate and adapt his diabetes management, and he is beginning also to contribute to local health planning decisions for diabetes patients.

In your clinical experience as a student nurse, you may have encountered examples of self-management that are based on the philosophy of the empowerment concept, for example patients with severe pain taking control over their pain management via 'patient-controlled analgesia' (known as PCA in surgical wards). This is a system whereby post-operative patients can self-control the dosage of analgesia they receive according to their pain levels by pressing a button that activates an electronically controlled pump to inject a prescribed opioid analgesic. Similarly, in the medical wards patients can self-administer their medication. Nurses play an active role in this, as each patient has to fulfil all the criteria for self-administration, as stated by local and national protocols. The nurse in collaboration with the patient reviews daily the self-management plan.

How empowered do you think patients feel? Do you think that patients have the same understanding of empowerment as health professionals? The case study evaluates the empowerment model of self-management very positively, with a high level of satisfaction and great enhancement of Robert's quality of life. This is very much in accordance with the literature, which reveals that empowerment benefits patients who are at the higher levels of the social spectrum.

We know that patients who are at a greater socio-economic disadvantage (read about inequalities in health in Chapter 6) tend not to be so empowered and are also less inclined to seek empowerment. The idea that the professionals know best, and that there is little the individual can do to help themselves, can be quite a barrier to developing self-management skills. To reach a level of critical consciousness may be a longer-term goal for these patients and therefore the nurses caring for them. Perhaps we need to think about a beginner level of health literacy at first (see Chapter 4).

Patient empowerment for people with long-term conditions imposes profound implications and challenges to nursing practice due to an already heavy workload, staff shortages and budget constraints that impede commissioning of self-management sessions. Nurses will need longer consultation periods to deal adequately with the demand of patient empowerment, both in a hospital or community setting (see Chapter 7). The NHS needs to put in place structures that facilitate a flow of communication and cooperative working practice between hospitals, primary care and social care and ensure a shared responsibility to meet the health needs of patients with long-term conditions.

Chapter summary

This chapter has enabled you to explore and develop your understanding of the need to support patients to self-manage their long-term conditions. It has also enabled you to use epidemiological evidence as a rationale to develop nursing practice that promotes patients' health and enhances their quality of life and to critically evaluate the

continued . . .

provision of health services to meet the health needs of patients suffering from long-term conditions by acting as the patients' advocate and challenging the political status quo. Your practice has to be informed by current health policy and apply the principles of the Expert Patient Programme, structured education programmes and empowerment. The chapter has encouraged you to evaluate critically their effectiveness, as well as to consider your changing role in your efforts to support patients to self-manage their chronic conditions.

Activities: brief outline answers

Activity 5.1: Critical thinking (page 91)

The list is not exhaustive. It may include: arthritis, asthma, chronic obstructive pulmonary disease (COPD), ulcerative colitis, Crohn's disease, diabetes (types 1 and 2), hypothyroidism, epilepsy, HIV/AIDS, Parkinson's disease, multiple sclerosis, cancers and mental health problems such as alcohol and substance abuse.

Many patients with long-term or chronic conditions have similar problems with:

- pain;
- limited mobility;
- sleep problems;
- depression;
- lack of social activities;
- difficulties with social support;
- eating or weight difficulties.

Activity 5.2: Reflection and critical thinking (page 97)

You may have found that the majority of them had similar views and needs, independent of their conditions.

- The majority of patients prefer to come to hospital only if it is absolutely necessary, in which case they would prefer it to be a planned admission.

- Most of the patients may have received health information from nurses and other health professionals on lifestyle issues, for example on exercise, diet or alcohol intake. Overall, patients want to have good, high-quality, simple information.

- They may want to have easy access to information to enable them to be more independent and pro-active about their self-care and management of their own health.

- Many may have expressed the need to have more support in the community, for example helplines (run by professionals specialising in their conditions) to seek support and advice as and when needed.

- They may want user-friendly and easily accessible NHS services, for example GP surgeries with longer opening hours.

Further reading

Department of Health (2007) *Supporting People with Long-term Conditions to Self Care.* London: DH.

This is a guide to supporting people with long-term conditions to self-manage through an integrated package that includes information, self-monitoring devices, self-care skills education and training, and self-care support networks.

Embrey, N (2006) A concept analysis of self-management in long-term conditions. *British Journal of Neuroscience Nursing,* 2(10): 507–13. Available online at www.internurse.com/cgi-bin/go.pl/library/article.cgi?uid=22535;article=BJNN_2_10_507_513

This is an analysis of the concept of self-management, theoretical but very useful in reviewing exactly what it entails.

The Health Foundation (2015) *A Practical Guide to Self-Management Support. Key Components for Successful Implementation.* London: The Health Foundation. Available online at: www.health.org.uk/sites/health/files/APracticalGuideTo SelfManagementSupport.pdf

This is a useful guide for all professionals involved in self-management support, as well as for patients to facilitate their self-management journey. It provides an overview of self-management support and identifies key components essential for a successful and effective implementation of self-management.

NHS Education for Scotland (2012) *Supporting People to Self-manage. Education and Training for Healthcare Practitioners: A Review of the Evidence to Promote Discussion.* Edinburgh: NHS. Available online at:https://www.chss.org.uk/documents/2014/03/supporting-people-self-manage.pdf

A comprehensive literature review of education and training for health practitioners to enable them to support people to self-manage their long-term conditions.

Useful websites

www.dafne.uk.com

This is the website of the DAFNE structured diabetes education programme.

www.desmond-project.org.uk

This is the website of the DESMOND structured diabetes education programme.

www.expertpatients.co.uk

This is the website of the Expert Patients Programme, a community interest company.

www.kingsfund.org.uk/projects/gp-inquiry/management-long-term-conditions

The King's Fund reports on its work on the management of long-term conditions.

www.nhs.uk/Planners/Yourhealth/Pages/Yourhealth.aspx

This is a guide for people with long-term conditions, giving lots of advice and practical information.

Chapter 6
Considering public health

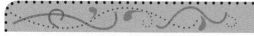

continued . . .

By the second progression point:

3. Understands the concept of public health and the benefits of healthy lifestyles and the potential risks involved with various lifestyles or behaviours, for example substance misuse, smoking, obesity.

18. Discusses sensitive issues in relation to public health and provides appropriate advice and guidance to individuals, communities and populations, for example contraception, substance misuse, smoking, obesity.

22. Works within a public health framework to assess needs and plan care for individuals, communities and populations.

Cluster: Infection prevention and control

21. People can trust the newly registered graduate nurse to identify and take effective measures to prevent and control infection in accordance with local and national policy.

By the second progression point:

6. Discusses the benefits of health promotion within the concept of public health in the prevention and control of infection for improving and maintaining the health of the population.

By entry to the register:

11. Recognises infection risk and reports and acts in situations where there is need for health promotion and protection and public health strategies.

Chapter aims

By the end of the chapter you will be able to:

- understand the scope of public health;
- describe the structure of public health functions in the UK;
- appreciate the role of the nurse in the control of communicable diseases;
- recognise the need to respond to public health emergencies.

Introduction

Public health is an overall term that covers aspects of disease prevention and health promotion, and is a broader term than treatments or care for people who are ill. Although much of what we do as nurses falls under the meaning of public health, it is not often recognised as such. Nurses get involved with preventing disease through immunisation and screening, but this is only part of their public health role. Their knowledge of the causes and population patterns of disease is helpful to nurses' understanding of why people become ill.

Most nurses, however, do not see themselves as public health practitioners. The NMC has set up a specialist register for nurses working in this area, which currently includes:

- health visiting;
- occupational health;
- school nursing;
- sexual health;
- health protection;
- family health nursing in Scotland.

The government intends to strengthen the public health function of nurses (DH, 2008a). You need to be aware that there is an increasing need for nurses to develop an understanding of and skills in public health practice even if you are not going to be on the specialist NMC register. In 2012 the Royal College of Nursing put out a position statement on nursing's contribution to public health, which states that *Regardless of the environments nurses work in or their titles or individual roles, all nurses have a part to play in improving the health of local people* (RCN, 2012, p3). Viv Bennett is currently director of nursing at the Department of Health and Public Health England; look out in the professional press for her news of what's happening in public health for nurses.

Outbreaks of various types of influenza and measles have shown that the public turn to nurses among other health professionals for reassurance and information. The current issue of children as young as 14 developing what used to be called elder-onset (type 2, non-insulin-dependent) diabetes should indicate to you that knowledge of disease causes and trends will help you understand and keep up with changes in healthcare practice.

What is public health?

On the one hand, 'public health' can be seen as a very general term to include all aspects of health – some writers use the term this way, which can be confusing. On the other hand, public health can be seen as everything except the treatment and care aspects of health – some writers use it to describe prevention of disease and promotion of health.

> **Concept summary: Definitions of public health**
>
> The usual definition in government documents and used by the Faculty of Public Health is: *the science and art of preventing disease, prolonging life and promoting health through the organised efforts of society* (Acheson, 1988).

The current public health white paper (DH, 2010b) also uses this definition and goes on to propose that the government expects the outcomes of public health practice to be in five areas (domains):

1. **health protection and resilience**: protecting people from major health emergencies and serious harm to health;

2. **tackling the wider determinants of ill health**: addressing factors that affect health and well-being;

3. **health improvement**: positively promoting the adoption of 'healthy' lifestyles;

4. **prevention of ill health**: reducing the number of people living with preventable ill health;

5. **healthy life expectancy and preventable mortality**: preventing people from dying prematurely.

Note that health promotion (quite commonly called health improvement) is a part of public health. Public health also addresses the factors causing disease and death.

Who does what in public health?

Each of the four UK countries has its own organisation for public health (see Useful websites at the end of the chapter). There have been various changes in recent years in the organisation names and responsibilities; follow the news in your country of practice to know who does what in public health.

There was a big change in England following the coalition government's 2010 white paper *Healthy Lives, Healthy People* (DH, 2010b) and the subsequent Health and Social Care Act of 2012. Along with other reforms, a major difference now is that the NHS continues to look after people who become patients, whereas health promotion/improvement in terms of public health generally is the responsibility of local government (local authorities/councils). They are supported by a ring-fenced public health grant and a specialist public health team, led by the director of public health. This is the work they do:

- health checks (four-yearly) of adults 40–74 – called the NHS Health Check programme;
- public health advice service – topics determined locally;
- health protection in local emergencies;
- weighing and measuring of children;
- sexual health services;
- general health improvement related to lifestyle issues – physical activity, healthy eating, drug and alcohol misuse, tobacco use, oral health behaviour and injury prevention.

Local authorities can commission these services from any qualified provider (AQP), including the NHS, following a tendering process based on quality and price.

Public Health England oversees the work of local authorities as well as managing national public health issues. Its priorities are to:

- reduce preventable deaths;
- reduce the burden of disease;
- protect the country's health;
- give children and young people the best start in life;
- improve health in the workplace.

Activity 6.1   *Critical thinking*

Go to the relevant public health organisation website for your country of practice and look up a topic that interests you. Have a look at the front page of the website for news first, particularly if there is a health crisis such as an epidemic or a heatwave happening at the time. Then use the site search engine to look up something either to do with your current practice area or to do with something you are curious about. Here are some suggestions:

- measles;
- campaigns for a specific time of year, for example Ramadan, or a specific topic, for example cancer;
- the new shingles vaccine;
- climate change;
- obesity;
- health checks.

There is no further guidance on this activity as it is to raise your interest in how public health works.

Main issues in public health

It is simpler to think of the work of public health professionals as divided into communicable (infectious, for example measles) and non-communicable (for example diabetes) disease prevention. They also seek to prevent harm from other less predictable occurrences, such as heatwaves, flooding affecting communities, radiation leaks and poisons. The WHO defines non-communicable diseases (NCDs) as *chronic diseases, which are not passed from person to person. They are of long duration and generally slow progression. The four main categories of noncommunicable diseases are cardiovascular diseases (like heart attacks and stroke), cancers, chronic respiratory diseases (such as chronic obstructed pulmonary disease and asthma) and diabetes* (www.who.int/mediacentre/factsheets/fs355/en – see this website for more information). Of course there are many other NCDs to think of, such as osteoporosis, depression or eczema.

For both communicable and non-communicable diseases it is possible to find statistics on epidemiology – the study of determinants (causes) and distribution (who gets the diseases and where) of each disease. This is called disease surveillance and it is carried out by the public health system. Doctors in general practice and in hospitals send reports of their diagnoses to the local directors of public health and the statistics are collated by the health observatories, which are able to help the health service plan for the future using the trends in diseases.

There are several ways to find health statistics:

- use the national statistics database available on www.ons.gov.uk – this website holds all national statistics on all topics including health;
- go to the website of your local community health organisation or local authority, as they have to produce an annual report on the health of their area;

- look at the local health profiles compiled by the public health observatories, available on www.apho.org.uk;

- if you want international statistics, use the WHO at www.who.int;

- use a search engine such as Google and type in the name of the disease you are interested in, plus the word 'statistics'.

Activity 6.2　　　　　　　　　　　　　　　　　　　　　　*Critical thinking*

Using one or more of the methods above, find statistics on two diseases – one communicable, for example chicken pox/shingles, and one non-communicable, for example bipolar disorder or stroke.

Find out who is affected more – some diseases will show greater demographic differences between:

- men and women;
- age groups;
- social classes or income levels;
- geographical locations;
- ethnic groups.

There is no further guidance on this activity as it is to raise your awareness of the availability of health statistics.

This activity should show you that with some diseases there are obvious differences. However, with others the differences may not be so obvious and the diseases are generally spread across the population.

In communicable diseases the rate and distribution of cases are related to how the infection has spread. This will not show up so much in statistical tables, but on maps and in the numbers of new cases occurring each day. NCDs can also be mapped, and may reveal the distribution of, for example, ethnic groups or families with very young children.

Communicable diseases

Case study: Outbreak of measles in Wales

An outbreak of measles in Swansea began in November 2012 with three cases notified. By the end of November it was clear there was an outbreak across schools in the Swansea area. Public Health Wales acted quickly to make the public aware of the risk to unvaccinated children. From April 2013, drop-in sessions for MMR (measles, mumps and rubella) vaccinations were held in GP surgeries, schools and hospitals in the area; 75,868 unscheduled vaccinations were given to people who had not been immunised.

---

continued . . .

The outbreak ended with the last case in May 2013. During that time there were 1,219 notifications of cases, 88 people needed hospitalisation and one young man died of pneumonia caused by the measles illness.

Public Health Wales (2013) has warned that unless MMR vaccinations continue, further outbreaks cannot be ruled out. The biggest group needing to 'catch up' are the 10–18 year olds, who missed out on their two doses in earlier childhood.

All epidemics of communicable diseases are tracked in the same way and nurses need to become aware of the public health actions taken. Your role in the circumstance of an epidemic such as this is to follow the story in the press and keep up to date with your employer's policies and procedures regarding the public health response.

Prepare yourself for your public health role so that you are able to:

- understand the risk of a person becoming infected;
- know the typical signs and symptoms;
- answer questions from patients, relatives and your local community about the risk;
- report promptly any relevant observations in patients (for example, raised temperature, rash) to nursing and medical staff;
- make sense of your employer's actions, such as immunisation of staff and closure of beds.

Activity 6.3   *Critical thinking*

Next time you read in the newspapers or see on the television that there is an outbreak of a communicable disease, follow the story in the press.

- Where and when did it start?
- How quickly is it spreading?
- Was it spread in a local area – how?
- Or was it spread globally by people travelling?
- How is the public responding? Is there panic, misunderstanding and confusion, or anger at a lack of information or action?
- What is the official information to the public?

There is no further guidance for this activity as it is to encourage you to follow a health story in the press.

As you become more aware of the public health aspects of communicable disease surveillance, you will see that some diseases seem to cause more alarm than others. Some are designated 'notifiable'.

Notifiable diseases

There are some communicable diseases that are considered to be very risky to populations and outbreaks need to be monitored and controlled quickly. Nurses need to be aware of these even though the notification is done mainly by medical practitioners. Doctors have to report cases of the notifiable diseases listed, to alert public health directors to possible outbreaks and epidemics.

Some of these diseases occur rarely and smallpox is an example of one deemed to be wiped out globally, but look at some of the commoner diseases on the list. You may come into contact with these, be asked by people for advice, or need to be on the lookout for potential cases in your nursing practice area. You can find the list of Diseases Notifiable (to Local Authority Proper Officers) under the Health Protection (Notification) Regulations 2010 on gov.uk/guidance/notifiable-diseases-and-causative-organisms-how-to-report

You will be aware, through the media, of 'new' communicable disease scares such as the Ebola and Zika viruses. People may ask you what to do about protecting themselves; they may be planning to travel to risky areas or are simply worried because of a lack of understanding. Your best resource is the NHS Health Choices website (www.nhs.uk) where you can find advice for these or other conditions. If possible, try to look at the site with the person asking you – teaching them how to find out for themselves.

As you will see, there are some very rare diseases on the list (for example, anthrax and plague), but also some that you are more likely to encounter (for example, measles and food poisoning). The public health actions for an outbreak of any of these diseases will be similar. You need to familiarise yourself with the signs and symptoms of the most common diseases, as well as the nursing actions to be taken and the immunisations recommended to prevent outbreaks.

Immunisation

Immunisation is a primary prevention measure for some communicable diseases. The UK has a schedule of immunisation for children, people at clinical risk and the elderly. This schedule is offered free through the NHS by health visitors and general practitioners. Local authorities work on behalf of the NHS in schools to immunise schoolchildren. Information for professionals and the public is available on the Department of Health website, www.dh.gov.uk

Look at the UK immunisation schedule online for the most recent version (www.gov.uk/government/publications/the-complete-routine-immunisation-schedule). Some of the most recent changes include a herpes zoster (shingles) vaccine for people in their seventies, annual influenza vaccine for children and a vaccine for rotavirus for babies. There is also a national catch-up programme for MMR vaccination to ensure all children (10–16) are covered, following a period when the vaccine was not taken up sufficiently in the late 1990s and early 2000s. Measles became a problem again due to the low vaccination level. A safe level for any community would 95 per cent.

This schedule is quite comprehensive but, as you will see, immunisation is recommended and made available but is not compulsory for UK residents. In some countries the public health authorities demand certain immunisations or make them compulsory for schoolchildren, immigrants and travellers.

People need to understand the importance of protecting themselves and their children from communicable diseases, and weigh this up against the perceived dangers of immunisation itself. They may also be unaware of the beneficial effects of having most of the population immunised, which is sometimes called 'herd immunity', when outbreaks are fewer and less severe if most people are immunised. The whole NHS, including nurses and other health professionals, is responsible for encouraging uptake of immunisations. In England since 2013, this has also become a part of the role of local authorities in promoting health, particularly targeting low uptake and hard-to-reach communities.

Activity 6.4　　　　　　　　　　　　　　　　　　*Communication*

Mr Watkins is 66 and has been advised by his GP to have the flu vaccine this year. Mr Watkins is worried that this will cause him to actually develop flu and he has heard stories about how it makes people feel unwell. He has also read that there are different types of flu and is puzzled as to how one vaccine could work for all of them.

- How will you put his mind at rest and how will you persuade him to take up the offer?

An outline answer is provided at the end of the chapter.

Working through this activity may help your own decision as to whether to take up the flu vaccine as a health professional. You too need to be protected.

Public health professionals worry about people not being immunised and about herd immunity. They monitor the uptake of immunisations and set targets for local community health organisations to achieve. For the flu vaccine, estimated uptake in those aged 65 years and over was 72.8 per cent (2009/10, 72.4 per cent); in the clinical risk groups under 65 years of age uptake was 50.3 per cent (2009/10, 51.6 per cent); and in pregnant women was 37.7 per cent as of 27 February 2011. As a country, despite our relatively high uptake by international comparisons, we have fallen short of the WHO aims. The UK current target for flu vaccine uptake is 75 per cent for people aged 65 years and over as recommended by the WHO; and 75 per cent for people under 65 with clinical conditions that put them more at risk from the effects of flu.

Some immunisations are even more contentious. Since September 2008 there has been a national programme to vaccinate girls aged 12 to 13, and to catch up with older girls aged 14 to 17, against the human papillomavirus (HPV), also known as the cervical cancer jab. The programme is delivered in secondary schools and consists of three injections that should ideally be given over a period of six months, although they can all be given over a period of 12 months.

Case study: The HPV vaccination

Mrs Foster, the wife of a patient on the surgical ward, asks a nurse for advice. She wants to know whether to allow her 14-year-old daughter to have the HPV vaccination. The nurse is interested

(continued)

---

continued . . . •

to know why Mrs Foster is questioning this as, in her view, the daughter should have all the protection she can get against cervical cancer.

The nurse sits down with Mrs Foster and asks her to say why she thinks the vaccination should not proceed. Mrs Foster says that she knows it's about a sexually transmitted disease and her daughter doesn't have sex. She fears the immunisation will make her daughter think about having sex when she is too young. Mrs Foster feels the school should not be allowing the issue of sex to be raised.

The nurse asks whether Mrs Foster has agreed to her daughter attending sex education classes at the school. She discovers that Mrs Foster has not withdrawn her daughter from classes (although she is entitled to); she has just allowed them to continue. The nurse continues to discuss the overall approach the school seems to have to sex education and states that, in her professional opinion, knowledge and understanding about sex is more likely to prevent early sexual experimentation than to encourage it. The nurse suggests that the HPV immunisation would raise further awareness of the risks of sexual intercourse and may deter her daughter from trying sex.

She goes on to explain that having the vaccination before sexual activity begins is more effective and it is the government's intention to create a general level of immunity in girls and young women. Mrs Foster agrees that it does, after all, seem a good idea and is pleased when the nurse gives her the website address for NHS Choices (www.nhs.uk) on which she can learn more about the HPV vaccine.

The role of health professionals in helping people to decide about immunisations is partly to allay fears that circulate in horror stories and rumour. We learned the lesson well from the problems caused by poor research into the MMR vaccine. Because of misleading research findings people became afraid of the effects of MMR, the uptake was poor and the result was low herd immunity resulting in several outbreaks of the diseases. Measles, in particular, is a disease that can kill, and children died in the outbreaks. Mumps in adults is more serious than in children (causing more severe symptoms and taking longer to recover from). The effect of not vaccinating with MMR for several years was that, when those unvaccinated children became adults at 18 and went to college and university, leaving home to live in community residences, outbreaks of mumps occurred in these places. As a nurse your opinion is respected by the public and it is important that you find out the facts and the best advice to give. MMR is safe and immunisation prevents communicable diseases; that is the message we should be giving the public.

Antimicrobial resistance

Moving now from primary prevention (immunisation) to tertiary prevention (preventing problems with treatment), the issue of failure to control infections because microbes become resistant to drugs is an increasing concern. Resistance arises because of several potential errors:

- Inappropriate prescription due to failure to follow guidelines – when antimicrobial drugs are given for the wrong organism (for example, antibiotics for viruses) or for self-regulating illnesses.

- Inappropriate prescription due to yielding to patient pressure or lack of time. Patients can be insistent when they think they need antibiotics.

- Patients failing to complete the course prescribed, so that effectiveness is lost and resistance develops.

There is guidance on Antibiotic Stewardship published by the National Institute for Health and Care Excellence (NICE) in 2015. The aim is to change prescribing practice as well as to inform the public (www.nice.org.uk/guidance/ng15). Nurses have a role in following the guidance, not only as a prescriber but also, perhaps, to discuss possible poor practice with other prescribers if you come across it. Another role is to teach patients and the public about the risks involved.

Having looked at a major part of what constitutes public health – communicable diseases – we will now return to an aspect of disease surveillance that appeared earlier but was not explored. In explaining what public health is we mentioned that the current white paper, *Healthy Lives, Healthy People* (DH, 2010b), includes 'tackling the wider determinants of ill health', and later in Activity 6.2 we asked you to look out for any differences in disease distribution due to 'social classes or income levels'. These allude to the issue of who is at more risk from ill health due to social rather than physical factors.

Inequalities in health

Concept summary: Health inequalities

Since the Black Report (DHSS, 1980) it has been known that social class impacts on health. Low socio-economic status (and particularly poverty) leads to a disproportionately high level of ill health. This was confirmed by Whitehead's work of 1988. Ignored or denied by the Conservatives, the issue was highlighted by the Labour government between 1998 and 2010. It commissioned the Acheson Report in 1998, which re-emphasised the fact that poverty and other social disadvantages affect health.

The current work on inequalities in health is informed by the Marmot (2010) review, which sets out six policy objectives:

- give every child the best start in life;
- enable all children, young people and adults to maximise their capabilities and have control over their lives;
- create fair employment and good work for all;
- ensure a healthy standard of living for all;
- create and develop healthy and sustainable places and communities;
- strengthen the role and impact of ill health prevention.

The history of the UK acknowledging and working on health inequalities originates in 1980 with the Black Report (DHSS, 1980) and shows how long the struggle has been to resolve these problems.

Inequalities in health are still a major government agenda today. The health of individuals and communities is greatly affected by social and environmental circumstances; the UK has poverty, poor housing, poor education, poor employment and social disadvantage today and public health continues to try to reduce these inequalities.

Working in partnership with other sectors such as housing, education and employment, public health and other health professionals seek to improve those social, economic and environmental circumstances that can trap people into cycles of disadvantage and therefore ill health. Improving health is not only about physical prevention such as immunisation, and not only about educating people about health: people need to be in better circumstances to have better chances of health.

Scenario: What caused the ill health?

Young Conan Smith (14 years old) is a traveller boy, one of seven children of Michael and Dawn, living on a caravan site on a wide road verge between two farms. He, his brothers and father do casual work on the farms during the fruit-picking season. His mother and oldest sister look after the van and the younger children. None of the children is going to school.

Conan had an accident while driving the tractor, badly lacerating his lower leg over the shin bone. He was not taken to hospital and has now developed a severe infection and is very unwell with a fever, loss of appetite and dehydration. His leg is not healing.

What are the causes of Conan's ill health?

Consider the scenario of Conan's ill health. The family background is one of a low level of education, imperfect housing, low income and poor use of health services. This leads to an inequality in health chances for traveller communities.

It is important to realise that in most Gypsy and traveller communities there are few problems of hygiene in the home and few problems of child neglect. The caravans are super clean (due to these communities' hygiene culture) and the children are loved and cared for. The hygiene problems come from a lack of toilet facilities and consistent water supply on the sites that they are forced to use. The discrimination and hate crime against the communities from local residents adds to the tendencies to violence, domestic disturbance and crime. Children are expected to grow up fast, often leaving school at 11 or 12, and working with the adults, marrying at 16 and setting up home for themselves. Boys in particular are expected to be strong, outgoing, protective of their families and not soft or needy in any way. There are problems with healthy eating in these communities, with a low intake of fruit and vegetables to aid growth and healing. There is a mistrust of health professionals and services and the care provided. In hygiene terms hospitals are seen as dirty because, for example, the separation of body washing and food serving is not good enough – think about the use of the bed tables for both functions. Vaccinations (tetanus in Conan's case) are also not trusted, and dressings on wounds are seen as unclean.

Health service provision is not geared up for traveller communities. People are expected to stay in one place for follow-up, for example. Schools provide health checks, but traveller children miss out because of moving frequently as well as leaving early. Educating these communities about health is essential but must be appropriate to their needs; for instance, with poor reading ability being common, leaflets are no use. Appropriate, culturally competent outreach programmes may be the answer.

Can you see from Conan's story how social, cultural, economic and environmental factors affect health?

Regulating for public health

Laws, policies and regulations in public health are used by government and local governments (through by-laws) to control the health environment for all people. There are many examples, such as seat-belt legislation, the ban on smoking, laws controlling recreational drugs, and local by-laws for behaviour in town centres. There are often economic considerations involved in monitoring (policing) and in larger effects on taxes and commercial interests. There are certainly ethical issues in controlling people's behaviour in this way, and one thing regulations don't do well is educate the people they are intended to control.

As an example, the coalition government of the UK intended, when it first came into office, to regulate for two particular behaviours:

- plain packaging on cigarettes (black lettering on white, no logos);
- minimum unit pricing on alcohol (not allowing cheap offers).

Both of these ideas were discussed in detail and supported by health professionals, including the Royal College of Nursing. The government retracted in spring 2013, on the basis of a lack of evidence of effectiveness, but some people believe that there was pressure from the tobacco and alcohol industries. There is an argument that such regulations would protect health, but others argue that there is no educative element and stigmatisation of consumers may result. Consider the idea of regulation being applied to other products, for instance plain packaging on junk food and minimum pricing of sunbed sessions. Similar arguments could be used.

One regulation that did get through the same session of parliament was putting in place a consistent nutritional labelling system on food products. The traffic light system had been proposed previously but was too inconsistently accepted by the food industry and retail supermarkets. In 2013, a standardised label was introduced that was more detailed and easier to interpret. This new label, instead of referring to the package (meal or snack) as a whole, breaks it down to labelling the fat, salt and sugar content separately. It makes it easier for people to tell if a package contains high (red), medium (amber) or low (green) fat, salt and sugar, also giving percentages. These front-of-pack labels provide people with more usable information to make choices (see Figure 6.1).

More recently, there has been further government regulation in tobacco and alcohol consumption to protect public health. Plain (or standardised) packaging for cigarettes was agreed to be introduced from May 2016. Packets show no brand colours or logos, and only state the brand and show text and pictorial evidence of the harm that smoking causes. In addition, there is new legislation regarding protecting children from second-hand smoke. It is illegal for drivers or

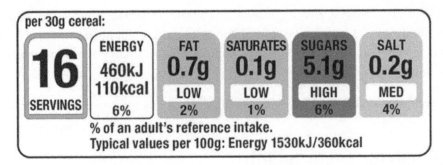

Figure 6.1: Front-of-pack labelling

passengers to smoke in a vehicle that is carrying someone under 18. Minimum unit pricing of alcohol has been discussed in parliament but no regulation has been made to date (Summer 2016). The issue is now further complicated by the decision to leave the European Union.

The question arises as to whether sugar intake should be regulated in order to prevent obesity and related health risks. The government has reviewed evidence to suggest that several actions would reduce sugar consumption, including controlling prices in shops and restaurants, banning advertising to children and regulating sugar content of food and drinks. The current advice is that sugar make up no more than 5 per cent (previously 10 per cent since 1991) of daily calorie intake – that is 30 grams a day. Find the rationale at www.gov.uk/government/publications/sugar-reduction-from-evidence-into-action. A new educational campaign was introduced in 2016 encouraging parents to get 'Sugar Smart' and take control of their children's sugar intake (more information on the website nhs.uk/change4life). However, the promised childhood obesity strategy was delayed several times, promoting speculation that there has been lobbying from the food sector. In the Budget of 2016, the government created a tax targeting drinks containing over 5 per cent sugar. Some public health activists believe this is inadequate and rather confusing since, for example, sugary milky drinks are excluded on the basis that milk is nutritious. Following this, the Childhood Obesity Strategy was published at last (HM Government, 2016b) to much criticism. Detractors declared it to be embarrassingly weak, throwing away the opportunity to make a real difference. Significantly the strategy fails to ban price-cutting of junk foods and fails to restrict advertising of foods high in salt, fat and sugar to children.

On the other hand, health improvement through public health measures raises some ethical issues around doing things to make people change their behaviour. For instance, the ban on smoking in enclosed public places removes some aspects of choice for smokers in the interests of enabling them to take the opportunity not to smoke.

> **Concept summary: Ethics in regulating for public health**
>
> Does regulating health behaviour remove *autonomy*? Consider the following examples:
>
> - making school meals compulsory;
> - limiting sales of alcohol;

(Continued)

- banning sugary drinks in schools;
- requiring children to be immunised;
- making spitting in the street a criminal offence;
- fluoridating water supplies;
- preventing advertising of snack foods to children.

Yes, these (some actual and some proposed) regulations mean the government is making decisions for people. So, could this be considered to be *beneficence* on the part of the government? Perhaps, because this type of regulation does good, whether the people like it or not! However, if a regulation is not based on sound evidence, the argument is lost and this may lead to mistrust.

What about *non-maleficence*? Could some regulations be seen to be doing no harm? On the one hand, perhaps food labelling is an example of a regulation that is helpful rather than harmful, and doesn't take away autonomous choice. On the other hand, requiring manufacturers to lower the levels of salt, fat and sugar in food products will do no harm, and may do some good, but takes away an element of choice (also it will not educate people).

Justice, as an ethical principle, is well served by public health regulation, because everyone would be treated the same. If drinking alcohol in the street is not allowed, then no one can drink in the street, which would be safer for all. As long as a regulation doesn't make life difficult for the disadvantaged in society, then it may be just. It also works the other way around; for those people considered to have inequalities in health, a regulation could even up their chances. If everyone were able to buy fresh fruit at controlled lower prices, families on lower incomes would benefit. Or would we want richer people to pay more?

As a nurse you need to be aware of public health regulations, both national and local, in order to answer patients' questions and to provide good practice and good care within legal frameworks. Keep up with the health news through the media; perhaps set up electronic news alerts, read newspapers and watch television news.

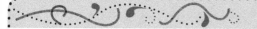

Chapter summary

This chapter has explored the meaning of public health and the nurse's role in the wider aspects of public health. You should now have a better understanding of the function of public health organisations and professionals. There has been a focus on communicable diseases in order to explain and help you understand your role, which is not what nurses think of every day as a nursing role. Inequalities in health have been introduced in order to help you envisage the whole picture of what causes ill health. The chapter has also explored some of the ethical arguments in controlling health behaviour through making regulations. As you continue to care for patients, you can consider the social, economic and environmental factors that brought them into your care.

Activities: brief outline answers

Activity 6.4: Communication (page 119)

The vaccine may cause Mr Watkins to feel a bit off-colour for a day but will not cause him to develop flu. While his immune system reacts to the vaccine his temperature may go up a little and he may feel sleepy and not want to eat because of this. The injection site may be very slightly inflamed. Any symptoms worse than this must be reported to his doctor, as he may have developed another infection while trying to respond to the vaccine.

He needs to know that it is better to be protected than to risk getting flu, which can be a severe illness, and may kill vulnerable people. The vaccine offered each year is the best available for the predicted outbreak that year.

Finally, tell him that if he has any fever or infection at the time of the appointment he must cancel or tell the nurse when he gets there. The immunisation should not be done when his immune system is fighting another infection, as he could become more ill – but he still would not get flu.

In addition, you must make sure that Mr Watkins is not immune-deficient because of cancer chemotherapy, organ transplant or HIV infection. This would mean that he only gets the flu vaccine under the care of his specialist experts.

Further reading

Coles, L and Porter, E (eds) (2009) *Public Health Skills: A Practical Guide for Nurses and Public Health Practitioners.* Oxford: Blackwell.

This is an edited book with chapter writers explaining a comprehensive range of skills for improving health in communities.

Useful websites

www.apho.org.uk

The Association of Public Health Observatories represents a network of 12 public health observatories working across the five nations of England, Scotland, Wales, Northern Ireland and the Republic of Ireland. They produce information, data and intelligence on people's health and healthcare for practitioners, policy makers and the wider community.

www.gov.uk/government/topics/public-health

This is the public health section of the Department of Health website. News will be on the front page, and recent documents are easily accessible. Use the search box to look up your topic.

www.ons.gov.uk/hub

This is the government's website for all UK statistics. Use the search box for the topic you need.
Finally, the websites for Public Health England, NHS Health Scotland, the Northern Ireland Public Health Agency and Public Health Wales are as follows:

www.gov.uk/government/organisations/public-health-england

www.healthscotland.com

www.publichealth.hscni.net

www.publichealthwales.wales.nhs.uk

Chapter 7
Managing health promotion in practice

NMC Standards for Pre-registration Nursing Education

This chapter will address the following competencies:

Domain 1: Professional values

5. All nurses must fully understand the nurse's various roles, responsibilities and functions, and adapt practice to meet the changing needs of people, groups, communities and populations.

Domain 4: Leadership, management and team working

7. All nurses must work effectively across professional and agency boundaries, actively involving and respecting others' contributions to integrated person-centred care. They must know when and how to communicate with and refer to other professionals and agencies in order to respect the choices of service users and others, promoting shared decision-making, to deliver positive outcomes and to coordinate smooth, effective transition within and between services and agencies.

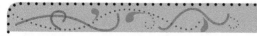

NMC Essential Skills Clusters

This chapter will address the following ESC:

Cluster: Organisational aspects of care

14. People can trust the newly registered graduate nurse to be an autonomous and confident member of the multi-disciplinary or multi-agency team and to inspire confidence in others.

By the second progression point:

 3. Values others' roles and responsibilities within the team and interacts appropriately.

By entry to the register:

 6. Actively consults and explores solutions and ideas with others to enhance care.
 7. Challenges the practice of self and others across the multi-professional team.
 8. Takes an effective role within the team adopting the leadership role when appropriate.
 9. Acts as an effective role model in decision-making, taking action and supporting others.
10. Works inter-professionally and autonomously as a means of achieving optimum outcomes for people.

Introduction

In the twenty-first century, nurses in their role as health promoters need to develop a health promotion practice that embraces the broader context of health, which includes the physical, psychological, socio-economic and environmental dimensions of well-being as discussed in Chapters 1 and 6.

In order to manage this practice, you need to adopt a systematic and structured approach to health promotion practice that expands beyond NHS boundaries. This means that you have to change your focus of practice and not think only of sick people but also of healthy people. You have to develop health promotion activity that does not focus exclusively on patients in a hospital setting, but that considers the whole population living in the community you serve and how to promote their well-being, which is sustainable within their own living and working environments. The WHO (1986) considers settings where people need health promotion to be where people live, work, play, learn, travel and love – so everywhere people are really. Could nurses be involved in all settings?

This chapter will explore where and how health promotion can be planned, and who can work together with nurses. It will look at the skills nurses need to plan and manage quality health promotion in hospital and with communities.

Understanding healthy settings in the context of your nursing practice

The WHO advocates that health promotion must take place within different settings, referred to as 'healthy settings', namely healthy schools, healthy universities, healthy hospitals, healthy workplaces and healthy neighbourhoods, to mention a few. The overarching aim is to target the whole population at the different stages of their life spans, for example children in schools, adults in their workplaces and everyone, including older people, in their neighbourhoods.

Nurses can work in a variety of such settings to promote well-being and positive health.

Concept summary: Health promotion settings for nurses

- NHS: NHS hospital trusts (adult nurses, mental health, children's nurses).
- NHS: local community health organisations (practice nurses, health visitors, district nurses, psychiatric community nurses and community nurses for learning disabilities).
- New in England: nurses working for local authorities as part of commissioned services for sexual health, smoking and adult health checks.
- Local education: schools, colleges, universities (school nurses, occupational health nurses).
- Local authority social care: residential homes, sheltered accommodation and nursing homes (adult nurses, mental health nurses, nurses for learning disabilities).
- Local authority with voluntary sector: neighbourhoods, housing estates, town centres, community centres, faith centres (health visitors, community nurses, nurses from all fields depending on speciality).
- Private sector: private hospitals, workplaces such as car manufacturing and department stores (occupational health nurses, nurses from all branches depending on speciality).
- Prisons (adult nurses, mental health nurses).

Settings such as these give nurses opportunities to develop health promotion activities suitable to the whole setting, not just to a particular target group on a particular health topic. Any one setting can include health promotion for everyone who is there (workers, visitors, students, patients, local families), on a range of topics such as coronary heart disease and cancer prevention, smoking, healthy eating, accident prevention, drug addiction, prevention of depression, and so on, whatever seems most relevant to the population of people you serve and your field of practice. This is a different approach to targeting groups and topics singly – for example, a teenage pregnancy project.

A setting is not only determined by its geography and the sector that finances the service provision. The WHO (1998) views a setting as the place in which people engage in daily activities such as working, learning, playing and loving. As a nurse you can identify with this concept of a setting, as it echoes the principles of the activities of daily living, which provides a familiar framework for your nursing practice. Alongside the daily activities you need to consider the setting's physical environment and infrastructure as well as people's personal factors, which interact to create and affect health and well-being. This means that you, as health promoter, have to view people (including patients) as part of the socio-economic context in which they live and to consider how this impacts upon their health (see Chapter 6). You will need to work out very carefully which framework of health promotion practice will be most appropriate for the setting in which you are going to deliver your health promotion interventions, for example you may use a behaviour change approach or an empowerment approach (see Chapter 2).

Therefore, from the health promotion perspective, it seems highly appropriate that the concept of healthy settings is widely used by different governments in their health policies to promote health:

- by solving health-related problems closer to their source;
- by recognising that the social, physical and economic environments form an integral part of people's health.

In 2016 the new *Leading Change, Adding Value* framework for nursing in England (Cummings, 2016) declared a commitment for nurses to work beyond traditional boundaries into 'place-based' (meaning settings) work to improve community health.

The healthy settings approach in health promotion practice has been built on a number of the WHO's charters and declarations (see Chapter 1), for example the Ottawa Charter (WHO, 1986), the Sundsvall Statement (WHO, 1991), the Jakarta Declaration (WHO, 1997) and the Bangkok Charter (WHO, 2005). All of them act as catalysts in adopting the settings approach as the way forward for health promotion practice. They highlight the importance of settings in the development and implementation of comprehensive health promotion strategies to improve people's health status and quality of life. They stress that promotion of health and well-being requires the creation of supportive environments, including not only healthcare settings but also places such as home, work and recreational facilities. They urge individual governments to invest in the provision of a settings infrastructure to promote health. In the UK this has materialised in the format of healthy hospitals, healthy universities, healthy schools, healthy workplaces and healthy neighbourhoods.

Healthy Cities (WHO, 1978) provided the blueprint for the implementation of the healthy settings approach to achieve health gain. The Healthy Cities programme uses health promotion interventions based on a social model responding to people's health needs as perceived and determined by them (felt, expressed and comparative), rather than on the 'normative' health needs determined by the professionals. It focuses on priorities for change as determined by the people and acknowledges that people's behaviour is shaped by the structural factors of their living environment.

However, you, as a health promoter, have to be aware that there are substantial differences between the different settings in relation to their organisational structure, ideological ethos as presented in the mission statements, culture and size, for example a hospital has a formal and hierarchical institutional culture in comparison with a residential care setting, which could be informal and more linear in structure. You need also to be aware that there are differences between the social contexts of settings belonging to the same sector, for example a school in an inner city has an inherently different social context from a school in a rural area.

These differences and the complexities of the settings within which people live their lives are very important, and you need to bear them in mind when you plan and deliver health promotion interventions. Your health promotion activities have to be relevant and tailor-made for your target group.

Case study: The varying needs and cultures of different target groups

Nurse Ryan is a specialist in sexual and reproductive health with a professional interest in family planning practice. She has been invited to deliver a session on sex education in two local comprehensive schools. The two schools have different social and cultural environments. School A is located in the poorest part of the local area, with high levels of diverse immigrant populations, while school B is situated in the most affluent part of the locality, representing mainly the indigenous population.

continued . . .

Nurse Ryan prepared the same content for both sessions. On the day of delivering the session she used a student-centred approach. Both sessions were very interactive and she felt that the students gained a lot from the sessions. However, she noticed that students' discussions in the two schools were differently focused. The students in the two schools were interested in different things.

School A students wanted to know more about fertility, as they were keen to have babies and had very romantic views of having intimate relationships. Many young girls perceived motherhood as the way forward as they were not too keen to continue with their education.

School B students were very keen to know about contraception, and the effectiveness and provision of contraceptive services. They were ambitious and wanted to further advance their education.

Both sets of students, though, were asking similar questions, for example regarding confidentiality issues and the availability of young people's clinics in their area.

This case study highlights that nurses have to adjust their practice to meet the needs of their target group and the cultural diversity of the setting. Culture can be viewed as an integral part of one's identity, shaped by different influences such as nationality, race, ethnicity, gender, social class, religion and language. It impacts on the way we think, communicate, interact with others and form our relationships. It is a powerful force on shaping our values and belief systems and our behaviour. Nurses must be culturally competent to deliver high-quality health promotion care regardless of people's cultural background or English language proficiency, in order to promote equity and healthy behaviours and improve **health outcomes**. The importance of developing **cultural competence** in practice has been highlighted by the WHO, the European Union and UK governments in their directives, health and social care policies and strategies. The NMC responded by integrating cultural competence into nursing curricula. However, within the field of healthcare provision cultural competence remains a challenging issue. Nowadays, the healthcare workforce is more **culturally sensitive** to the health needs of multicultural Britain; however, patients from ethnic minorities still have difficulties in accessing appropriate healthcare due to language barriers and having different perspectives on health and expectations about treatment (see Chapter 3 on screening.) Policy makers, healthcare providers and healthcare systems need to integrate a multicultural approach to meet the health needs of the changing multicultural demography of the UK.

You can achieve cultural competence for health promotion practice by being willing and motivated to develop the following.

- **Cultural awareness**: through reflection you need to recognise and master personal prejudices, assumptions and stereotypical views about people from different backgrounds from your own. Self-awareness will enable you to organise and deliver a non-judgemental and anti-discriminatory health promotion practice.
- **Cultural knowledge**: striving to obtain and expand cultural knowledge to enhance your understanding about different cultural values and beliefs, customs and health perceptions. Processing and integrating this knowledge into your practice will ensure that your practice

is tailor-made to meet the **affective** needs of culturally diverse populations. An example will be to use drama or dance as a health education medium to increase breast awareness for Asian women.

- **Cultural skills**: this can be twofold – an ability to collate evidence-based cultural epidemiological and demographical data when you consider provision of health promotion services (for example, sickle cell screening and genetic counselling); and an ability to carry out culturally appropriate health assessments and perform sensitive clinical examinations (for example, health education for healthy nutrition or performing cervical screening for Muslim women).

- **Cultural encounters**: engagement in cross-cultural interactions by encouraging integration rather than segregation, for example promoting engagement in multicultural physical activity projects.

In summary, a settings approach challenges nurses to take the lead to improve the health status of the whole population rather than people who are ill. You have to develop skills in managing health promotion practice and to establish networking as well as to form partnerships (see Chapter 1). This means that you as a health promoter need to expand the horizon of your activities and to reconsider the nature of your practice, both of which will be discussed in the following sections.

Health promotion practice within an NHS setting: hospital and community

NHS Hospital Trusts and **NHS local community health services** are in a strong position, as settings, to provide health promotion, as they have professional expertise and captive target groups (staff, patients and visitors). Staff are generally well respected and valued by the public, and therefore they are seen as credible sources for health information and consultation.

Currently, the majority of nurses working within an NHS setting are involved with health promotion activities focusing on solving health problems, as presented by individual patients, and therefore the focus of their health promotion is oriented around disease prevention and management of disease. The activity constitutes part of the care plan documentation and is mainly delivered in the format of tertiary prevention (treatment and rehabilitation), health advice (see Chapters 1 and 4) and behaviour change (see Chapter 2).

One may argue that tertiary prevention is more typical of the health promotion work of nurses working within the hospital setting, than of nurses working in the primary care setting. Nurses in primary care have a wider scope of health promotion activity than hospital nurses as they are engaged, for example, in primary prevention such as vaccination and immunisation programmes, and secondary prevention such as screening, health checks and travel health services. However, health advice and behaviour change are needed in both sections of the NHS.

Nurses in NHS healthcare settings encounter many competing factors that constrain health promotion activities, for example clinical and care management issues, staffing levels and workload. As a result, health promotion is very often unplanned and opportunistic in nature, which can be effective, but more could be achieved if health promotion was integrated within the organisation and delivery of care.

Whether a hospital or community care area is committed to improving and maintaining good health promotion practice depends to a large extent on the vision and skills of its senior nurses. You may see areas that are doing some of the following, for example:

- planning calendar health events, such as Breast Cancer Awareness Month, No Smoking Day, HIV/AIDS and sexual health week, etc. – health events aim to encourage people to stay healthy as well as to change behaviour;

- making available health promotion leaflets relating to health topics of their specialty as a resource accessible to staff, visitors and patients;

- ensuring that every patient receives a health education programme that is standardised and recorded within the nursing care 'package';

- designating one qualified nurse as 'health promotion nurse' for the area, to coordinate activities and keep everyone else aware of the need.

As a qualified nurse you will need to become a catalyst for change by promoting and developing a practice within the NHS that is driven by national and international health strategies. If the organisation you work for does not have a strong and sustainable health promotion practice, be bold enough to suggest how they can improve. Start small in a small area or with one topic and care group, but go ahead and try something!

However, it has to be acknowledged that this can only be achieved by you developing competencies and skills to undertake the management of health promotion projects, by becoming a self-confident, knowledgeable practitioner with special expertise in health promotion, a political player and an active as well as influential participant in decision making at the organisational level. At present nurses are seen as 'doers' at the grass roots (micro) level rather than as initiators of change, and active participants in the decision making at a higher organisational (macro) level. As a graduate nurse, you will need to assert yourself in a leadership position regarding health promotion practice and to possess negotiation skills in order to gain the organisation's management support for funding, and to develop collaborative action. Planning, implementation and evaluation have to be the steering forces of managing health promotion practice at micro or macro level.

Managing health promotion practice in any setting requires a wide range of skills. Some of them are transferable skills from your nursing practice, for example interprofessional working, communication, planning, implementing and evaluating practice, as you will find out by doing Activity 7.1.

Activity 7.1   *Critical thinking and reflection*

You are working in a GP surgery as part of your clinical experience. The local community health organisation for the surgery, in collaboration with the local hospital, which has been awarded a healthy hospital status, has gained funding to develop a three-year programme with the aim of improving the quality of life of people who suffer from mental health problems in the local area. Your designated mentor, Theresa, has been given the remit to develop this programme. Theresa decides that the target group will be unemployed people who are known to be at risk of mental health problems. Theresa's objectives are:

- to set up a support group to enable them to come to terms and cope with their personal problems;
- to establish a drop-in centre that is easily accessible.

When Theresa discussed with you the proposed development, you expressed interest and volunteered to shadow Theresa during the developmental process of the programme. Now make a list of the skills you think Theresa will use during the planning process.

An outline answer is provided at the end of the chapter.

Reflecting on the activity, you may have identified a number of transferable skills from your nursing practice or your previous experiences; however, you may have encountered some difficulty in translating them into health promotion practice suitable to the setting, as well as into your role as an enabler, mediator and advocate of patients.

The organisation Skills for Health was tasked in 2004 with generating a list of skills for public health at specialist and practitioner levels. Specialists are professionals who are in charge of public health locally and nationally, and who act to manage public health locally and control emergencies (see Chapter 6). Public health practitioners can be from a variety of professions whose job includes working on improving health. This includes nurses on the NMC public health part of the register (see Chapter 6). Since the original listing of skills there have been several revisions and expansions. On the website for Health Careers (www.healthcareers.nhs.uk/about/resources/public-health-skills-and-knowledge-framework) you will find a long list of skills and knowledge at various levels to identify your development. Here is short version to consider now. You may like to refer back to this section when you have read Chapter 8 about keeping up your skills.

Concept summary: Skills and knowledge for public health

1. Surveillance and assessment of the population's health and well-being
- Being able to understand how health data are collected, interpreted and used to assess the health needs of people and communities.

(Continued)

2. Assessing the evidence of effectiveness of interventions, programmes and services to improve population health and well-being

- Review the literature and appraise evidence.

3. Policy and strategy development. Developing quality and risk management within an evaluative culture

- Interpret local and national policies, guides, etc. and implement in practice.

4. Leadership and collaborative working for health and well-being

- Appreciating that working in partnership with people and organisations to set up health promotion (interprofessional, interagency and intersectoral) is complex and can be effective.

5. Health improvement learning

- How to provide health information that is appropriate and relevant to people and communities, and helping them to change to healthy behaviour.

6. Health protection

- Recognising health risks and reducing health inequalities.

7. Public health intelligence

- Interpreting health statistics and data.

As with your nursing practice, you need to consider how you are going to find evidence of good practice in health promotion, which will inform your own practice and can be replicated in your setting. For example, imagine that you are planning to implement the National Service Framework for Diabetes (DH, 2001) to promote healthy drinking for your diabetic patients. You need to do a literature review to establish the effectiveness of similar projects and to review how others have set up the projects. You may also need to use epidemiological evidence to support and justify the need for such a project in your setting. Good IT skills and knowing how to conduct a literature search are crucial. Use different search engines as sources, for example MEDLINE, the Cochrane Database of Systematic Reviews, DARE (Database of Abstracts of Reviews of Effects) and the EPPI-Centre's database of reviews of effectiveness in health promotion.

Once you have read the gathered literature you need to critically analyse the material and to consider selection of health promotion interventions appropriate for your own setting. Many students find it difficult to analyse read material (literature). An easy way to achieve this is by considering yourself to be a good detective. Be inquisitive and always ask yourself: What does this mean for my practice? What are the implications for my practice? You need to translate the meaning of what you have read and to make judgements of read material in relation to quality, relevance, applicability and implications for your practice.

Identification of health needs enables you to set health promotion priorities, encourages patients' participation and promotes a health promotion practice that is patient-centred; therefore it is pertinent that you understand the hierarchy of needs. Bradshaw's taxonomy (Bradshaw, 1972) gives you a useful classification of needs that can guide your practice.

Concept summary: Bradshaw's taxonomy of needs

1. Normative needs
These are determined by professionals; for example, you as a nurse made the decision that diabetic patients need to have health education on foot care. The need represents your professional judgement and does not represent your patients' wishes. This is a top-down approach and does not take into account your patients' personal circumstances or factors, which may interact with their diabetes and affect their overall health and well-being. Health promotion takes the form of information giving and it very often reduces patients' concordance.

2. Felt needs
These are what your patients actually want. In the case of your diabetic patients, they may want better services and easier access to chiropodists. This allows for a bottom-up approach and you may act as a mediator to improve chiropodist services in the setting. However, you need to be aware that felt needs are based on individual perceptions and your patients may not actually be aware of the available chiropodist services in the locality, in which case you then provide information regarding access and availability of services.

3. Expressed needs
These are 'felt' needs turned into action and therefore have become a demand. Your diabetic patients are complaining about the prolonged waiting times to see a chiropodist in their locality. You need to be cautious that quite often the expressed needs represent the patients who are articulate and have the power and ability to make their voices heard. There is a danger that the most 'needy' may not express their needs and therefore health inequalities persist.

4. Comparative needs
These occur when a group of diabetic patients does not receive any health promotion activity in relation to foot care, while another group, which is similar in characteristics and of a similar setting, receives health promotion regarding diabetic foot care. This has been highlighted in relation to the so-called postcode lottery, where patients, depending on where they live, may or may not have access to certain treatments, for example NHS fertility treatment.

A skilful assessment, clear understanding and correct interpretation of health needs enables you, as health promoter, to set health priorities that represent the actual health needs of the setting's population, and you can plan appropriate and relevant interventions that will determine successful and positive outcomes of practice. You need to be aware that normative needs inform most health promotion activity in an NHS hospital ward or local community health setting, while felt and expressed needs will often be the guiding force in community development, which is usually operated in partnership with the community.

You need to be skilful in identifying the views of stakeholders. They are the people in the setting who have a vested interest in the health promotion project (for example, managers or budget holders) and they want to influence the 'what and how' of your health promotion practice. You need to pay attention to their views as they are in a position of power. However, you will need to establish that they do not compromise the calibre and overall purpose of your practice. This is very difficult to achieve and requires very skilful negotiation.

You need also to consider your target group, who are the recipients of the project. You need to pay attention to their values, beliefs, behaviour patterns, customs and culture, aspirations and attitudes. Your practice has to consider all these elements in order to be accepted by your target group.

This means paying attention to conflicts of interest between stakeholders and target groups and how these impending tensions may affect your practice within the setting. You need to be confident and assertive, have self-esteem and be an effective communicator and counsellor.

You need to develop a clear understanding of underpinning communication theories and to evaluate their merits (see Chapters 2 and 4). This will enable you to use a range of approaches to support people and facilitate change by promoting health-enhancing relationships that increase self-esteem and improve self-concept (see Chapters 1 and 2). By using the right language and by demonstrating understanding of their individual settings, you will be able to gain their cooperation. They will be motivated to engage in decision making. They will feel comfortable to seek support when they encounter difficulties.

The success of your practice depends on your management skills: you will need to employ a variety of management skills in order to develop a health promotion practice.

- You will need to be able to manage change, for example from what is done currently, which may be unplanned and under-resourced, to a formal, structured and well-organised practice.

- You have to be diplomatic, involve your colleagues in the decision-making process, gain their cooperation and be careful not to alienate them!

- Team building skills are crucial, as coordination and team work are vital. Health promotion practice involves working with people from different sectors and different departments. Therefore, it is vital to promote team building to maintain good relationships.

- Time management skills are very important and very difficult to achieve, as you may have already experienced while studying on the nursing degree course. As a nurse working in a very busy setting you are involved with a wide range of work roles, all of which compete for your time. You need to devise a realistic work schedule and ensure adherence to the schedule.

- You will need to seek management's support and approval, and secure their commitment to your practice. Negotiation skills will be helpful here.

- You will select a wide spectrum of resources for your practice (human and material). Critical review of various resources is an important element. You have to develop expertise in establishing their effectiveness, appropriateness and accessibility. You have to ask such questions as: Do they use clear language suitable for my target group? Are they non-racist, non-sexist? Are there any legal issues regarding consent? What is the evidence of their effectiveness? Who are the authors? What are their qualifications and expertise on the subject matter? Do they promote the interest of any particular party? See Chapter 4 for more details on choosing resources.

- Your role as health promoter also requires you to become an active networker and effective collaborator. High-quality collaborative action and skilful networking can be instrumental to successful, effective and efficient health promotion practice. This requires development of organisational, social, political, interpersonal, negotiation and leadership skills. In an NHS setting nurses, as patients' advocates, mediators and enablers, have to take the lead in forming partnerships (see Chapter 1). The partnership has to incorporate professionals drawn from the broad spectrum of the setting's multi-disciplinary team, such as doctors, physiotherapists, managers, specialist nurses, social workers and health promotion specialists, as well as external agents such as pharmaceutical companies.

- Your health promotion practice in an NHS setting will involve the development of a project or a programme, which is informed by national health policies and, as such, is funded by central government. However, very often you may be involved with local initiatives and, as such, you have to raise additional funds from other sources, for example the National Lottery. Thus you need to develop skills in writing proposals and presentation skills to secure funding for the project/activity, and the ability to use spreadsheets to estimate and monitor costs.

As a nurse already, you have the acquisition of planning, implementing and evaluating skills through the nursing process and will be able to transfer them to health promotion practice.

You need to assert your health promotion role by readdressing your scope of practice from an opportunistic, unplanned mode of practice to a well-thought out scheduled practice underpinned by the theoretical principles of planning, implementation and evaluation. Health promotion is frequently criticised for its lack of evaluation. Nowadays, working in an economic climate of austerity, you need to provide evidence not only of an effective and efficient practice, but of a health promotion practice that has an economic, social and health impact. This can be achieved by the process of evaluation.

Project planning

Activity 7.2	*Critical thinking*

As a graduate, you are the designated nurse for health promotion in an acute medical ward. The ward manager during a ward meeting reported that, according to the admissions

continued . . .

statistics, there was a marked increase in hospital admissions due to testicular cancer. During the meeting it was agreed that you should organise a health event in the main part of the hospital to promote awareness of testicular cancer among staff, patients and visitors.

• Think how you will plan, implement and evaluate the 'event'.

An outline answer is provided at the end of the chapter.

Chapter 1 offers some theoretical frameworks, for example Tannahill (1985) and the revised Tannahill (2009) model of health promotion, which help you to understand the nature and intention of health promotion practice. They also enable you to select and use appropriate interventions to improve the health of your patients – in Tannahill's model, education, prevention and policy. However, such frameworks do not give you a clear direction on the 'know how' to structure and manage your practice. Project-planning processes are helpful here. These consist of different well-defined stages that echo the nursing process, that is, the planning, setting goals, implementing and evaluating process. The process provides you with a series of linear stages that relate to each other and are cyclical in nature. They are very easy to follow and, by the application of relevant skills, as discussed in this section, enable you to organise and manage your health promotion practice.

Concept summary: Project-planning process

1. Assess needs and priorities.
2. Set aims and objectives.
3. Decide the best way of achieving the aims and objectives.
4. Identify resources.
5. Plan evaluation methods.
6. Set an action plan with details, dates and who does what.
7. Action! Implement your plan, including your evaluation.
8. Compile a report for the organisation and for your portfolio.

These stages provide a framework for practice that is already familiar to you and forms an integral part of your organisation of nursing care. They effectively enable you to incorporate health promotion as part of your nursing practice. This process can be applied to individual patient care also, and therefore the 'patient teaching process' can run parallel to the nursing process in operation. As a means of planning an independent project, however, it is a systematic approach to work and, as such, will be helpful to you whenever you want to introduce some new initiative into your practice.

Case study: Project planning

(Numbers relate to the project planning process in the concept summary above.)

Amina is a nurse working in an Accident and Emergency (A&E) department of a busy acute hospital Trust. She has been asked by her manager to join the multi-disciplinary planning team working on raising alcohol awareness. The decision to focus on alcohol has been influenced by increasing rates of alcohol-related admissions (accidents on the road and in the home, fighting outside the pubs, sexual assaults in the park and domestic violence) (1). A&E departments across the UK are keen to reduce admissions and to get the message across about the dangers of alcohol misuse (2). The team discusses targeting the local high street, which is not traffic-free and has three pubs, the main gate to the park and the local library. It is thought that people would receive health messages about alcohol more readily in familiar local venues (2).

While some other members of the team form a sub-group to plan joint work with the police on Friday and Saturday nights (3), Amina suggests working with the local library to get the message across. She visits and talks to the local librarians to discuss setting up displays, using the computer training sessions and arranging open events (3). After the visit she searches online for organisations to help, and finds Change4Life, Drink Aware and Alcohol Concern, who may join in events or provide health education materials (4). She also decides to produce a leaflet herself, detailing the link between drinking to excess and the local A&E experience – the team thinks this is a good idea and everyone wants to have an input (4). The librarians suggest that their literacy and computer training sessions with the public could use some of the online and printed materials Amina has found (4). In her investigations Amina makes contacts among her professional colleagues who agree to help at events such as displays and talks in the library (4).

In order to evaluate the effectiveness of her library initiative, Amina decides that there will be short questionnaires and a collection box at the displays and events. The intention is to find out what people find useful, whether they think anything else is needed and whether they take materials home to read and pass on to family members (5). Amina plans to go back after a month to talk to the librarians and ask them their opinions too (5). Before she started, Amina set out a time chart of tasks to do herself, including time to visit the library, to find resources, to design the evaluation questions and also decide on potential dates for displays and events (6). Later she was able to fill in this chart with actual planned tasks, recording when they were completed (7).

Finally, Amina designs a format for a report that complements the effectiveness measures being used by the whole team, including numbers of people attending and costs of the project (8). This library work report is later included in the main report to the hospital Trust and all partners in the initiative.

Partnership working: interprofessional, interagency and intersectoral

Nurses are not the only people who do health promotion as part of their role. Other health professionals all have the responsibility to teach patients and to contribute to health promotion initiatives.

You will find that hospital-based health professionals tend to concentrate on teaching patients as hospital nurses do, and community professionals tend to be the ones to work on wider projects.

The term 'agency' refers to the different organisations that exist in all aspects of the community. The GP practice and the sexual health clinic working together are two agencies within the NHS. The specialist colorectal nurse and the charity Beating Bowel Cancer, with which he or she is working, are also two agencies, this time across two sectors: public (NHS) and voluntary (charity). Different health professionals, different agencies and different sectors working together will all have their primary functions and unilateral ways of doing things. The primary function of a catering company is to sell food, so will they agree to your healthy eating advice in your project? The potential breadth of partners across professions, agencies and sectors can be large and at times clumsy. The various power levels of partners can get in the way of joint working. When partnership is effective, however, it can form a useful range of expertise and resources, and can be a powerful force for change. Activity 7.3 asks you to consider this breadth and will make you think about the skills you will need to communicate, network and manage a team.

Activity 7.3   *Team working*

You are working in the community with a community mental health nurse who has decided to set up an awareness-raising event in the local community centre. There has been an increase in the number of children diagnosed with depression locally, particularly children of families living in known deprived areas. The local people are a mixture of several cultures, some of which have a limited knowledge and acknowledgement of mental illness, especially in children. There is generally a low level of understanding of parenting skills.

At an informal meeting with the local GP practice team, you are asked to contribute to a brainstorm on who can be involved in this event.

- What ideas can you think of across the health professions, agencies and sectors?

An outline answer is provided at the end of the chapter.

From this activity you can see the possible range of help available through working in partnership to do health promotion. It is a time-consuming and complex way to work, but an enriching experience essential to a settings-based approach.

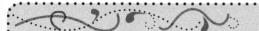

Chapter summary

This chapter has taken the issue of managing health promotion in practice and examined this in the context of healthy settings, skills for health promotion, planning projects and working in partnership. It has perhaps stretched your thinking further than the context of your student nurse role and experiences, but intends to show you the potential of your health-promoting role.

Activities: brief outline answers

Activity 7.1: Critical thinking and reflection (page 134)

Theresa will use a range of skills as specified by Skills for Health (2004).

- Collection of epidemiological data to ascertain the scale of the problem, that is, how many unemployed people live in the area and what are the rates of mental health problems among unemployed people?
- Communication with the unemployed and some key health professionals about the project, and assessing health needs.
- Doing a literature search for evidence and examples of best practice.
- Understanding local policies on mental health and knowing the local facilities.
- Assessing resources required for the project and securing funding.
- Setting up a team or teams; identifying and managing interprofessional working.
- Organising a work schedule.
- Leading the work of teams to achieve the project's objectives.

You may have noted other skills, such as the transferable skills of communication, IT skills, team work, or things such as writing skills and planning skills. The idea is that many skills are needed for this complex task.

Activity 7.2: Critical thinking (page 138)

- Create a time schedule – time for event preparation, fixing the date, evaluation of the event, writing up and publication.
- Form partnerships with other professionals who can contribute and participate in the organisation of the event (internal and external to the hospital), organise meetings, agree tasks, divide up the work and arrange staffing for the event.
- Set and agree aims and objectives for the event.
- Contact UK cancer and men's health organisations for current health information and promotion material, such as posters, leaflets, DVDs, models and illustrations of the body parts and quizzes on the facts.
- Order and review the resources; organise the venue and think about the layout of the display.
- Complete a health and safety risk assessment regarding venue and event.
- Discuss how you are going to approach the public and engage them in conversation.
- Design the event advertising and market the event. Remember you need to invite visitors, patients and staff.
- Plan the day – start and finish times, and who will set up and clear away. Organise tasks for each helper and a work schedule including coffee breaks.
- Keep a record of how many people came to the event, how many leaflets they took and how many participants completed quizzes. Ask people to write down what they thought of the event.
- Arrange a debriefing meeting with partners and ascertain how they felt the day went.
- Write an evaluative report of the event and publish internally or externally.
- Make an entry in your professional portfolio.

Activity 7.3   *Team working (page 141)*

You may have other ideas – but here are a few potential partners:

- GPs, practice nurses, social workers and school nurses;
- local community and hospital mental health services;
- youth workers, school counsellors, and relevant clinical psychologists and psychiatrists;
- locally involved YMCA, scouts/cubs, guides/brownies, sea cadets and any other local groups;
- Royal College of Psychiatrists, MIND, Depression UK, Kids Helpline, Young Minds, the Mental Health Foundation and the Depression Alliance;
- local faith group leaders, parents (perhaps there is a school group, or local estate group), and some of the children who have recovered;
- parenting skills teachers, and local library staff to continue the resource management.

There are guidelines on depression in children and young people from the National Institute for Health and Care Excellence (NICE), produced in 2005 – http://guidance.nice.org.uk/QS48. These have been followed up with quality standards in 2013 – http://guidance.nice.org.uk/CG28.

Further reading

Coles, L and Porter, E (eds) (2009) *Public Health Skills: A Practical Guide for Nurses and Public Health Practitioners.* Oxford: Blackwell.

This is an edited book with chapter writers explaining a comprehensive range of skills for improving health in communities.

Goodman, B and Clemow, R (2010) *Nursing and Collaborative Practice.* Exeter: Learning Matters.

This is a good book on collaboration and team work.

Verzuh, E (1999) *The Fast Forward MBA in Project Management.* Chichester: Wiley.

This is a very comprehensive and detailed guide to managing projects in any area. It has many ideas for organising effective teams and achieving outcomes.

Useful websites

www.uclan.ac.uk/research/explore/themes/healthy_settings_unit.php

This is the UK Healthy Settings Unit, based at the University of Central Lancashire. It is the place to find out what settings are used here, and the news about them.

www.who.int/healthy_settings/en

This is the WHO's site for healthy settings of all kinds across the world.

Chapter 8
Keeping up your skills

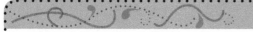

Introduction

This chapter focuses on keeping up your skills for health-promoting nursing practice. It considers the importance of understanding the guidance from the NMC with regard to **continuing professional development**. There is a variety of ways you may wish to keep up to date in health promotion practice and some suggestions are presented. It is also important to consider how you will collect the evidence of this work you have undertaken; this will be needed to underpin your professional practice.

Developing health-promoting practice skills

Today's NHS is going through a period of immense change. Nurses are learning new skills and playing a more active role in managing people's health and well-being, both in hospital and in the community. Developing the skills of being an effective health-promoting nurse in your workplace is a demanding but satisfactory area of your practice. The best way to become a health-promoting nurse is not to think that you have to make extra time to 'carry out' health promotion; rather, you should adopt a way of practice that makes health promotion rooted in the goals and outcomes and the environment of everyday work, at the same time encouraging others to join in. For example, there will be a 'culture' in everyday practice in the workplace for infection control, so similarly develop a 'culture' for health promotion practice among your colleagues.

The people you meet in your day-to-day practice will have expectations of the care and support for their problem of the moment. They should also be able to expect that you will take that help forward to support their future well-being with health-promoting practice. To be an effective health-promoting nurse involves, as indeed do all areas of practice, updating personal learning and being aware of why and how we go about this.

Continuing professional development

Continuing to keep skills updated, in order to learn and extend knowledge for practice, is expected of all nurses throughout their working lives (NMC, 2015). The NMC states that the people in your care must be able to trust you with their health and well-being; further, that you provide a high standard of practice and care at all times. Effective from March 2015, the NMC code reflects the world in which we live and work and has four themes:

- prioritise people;
- practise effectively;
- preserve safety;
- promote professionalism and trust.

Nurses must therefore make time to keep updated with new developments and research within public health and health promotion in order to be well informed about their practice. At university, as a student, goals for learning and practice have been structured and organised for you. In the future as a qualified nurse you will find that you will have the responsibility for your own learning and updating your practice. If you have developed good study habits and regularly set aside time for updating and reading, you will find it easier to find the time to continue such professional development activity as you become qualified. Continuing professional development has important implications for accountability to the public. Recipients of care have a right to access practitioners who possess up-to-date knowledge, skills and abilities appropriate to their sphere of practice. This book has suggested that nurses need to address the health promotion needs of their patients wherever care is given. Further, as the development and complexity of organisations continues to grow, there is demand for wider ranges of skills from practitioners. Nurses must therefore be prepared to develop and expand their health-promoting skills.

Thinking about health promotion

Effective health promotion and public health updating can involve several activities or elements of personal learning, such as being aware of public health at a strategic level (see Chapters 3 and 6). It can also be at a more immediate level in day-to-day encounters with patients (see Chapters 2 and 5). Whatever the level, being aware of recent developments is essential for ensuring that the best possible practices for health promotion are used (NMC, 2015). The Department of Health and organisations such as the NHS and NICE are sources of public health-related news, as are organisations such as the British Heart Foundation and Diabetes UK. It is always a good idea to check their websites for recent news and updates, remembering to put in the details of the health topic for the immediate guidelines or update available. For example, you can check the NHS guidance for seasonal flu on www.nhs.uk/conditions/Flu/Pages/ Introduction.aspx, or the up-to-date guidance on national campaigns such as skin health and sun exposure at the British Association of Dermatologists on www.bad.org.uk.

Professional development learning can happen very quickly during your practice experiences. Student nurses are advised to use reflection and to collate and analyse their learning, in order to be able to inform future practice. Health promotion practice forms part of this learning curve. Confidence in this area of practice comes from exposure to as many situations as possible, learning from patients and their families, even perhaps being on the receiving end of NHS healthcare yourself as a consumer.

You can think of your practice and reflection by thinking of Tannahill's model of health promotion practice and thus structure your reflective writing. It is also good to incorporate the new code themes.

Concept summary

Example 1: Health protection and reflecting on Continuing Professional Development (CPD).
Reading and updating on the new healthy eating plate guidelines.

> As a nurse I understand that this is essential knowledge for ensuring a nutritious balance for patients in my care and upon discharge.

> I will observe what the patients eat and that they understand what is a good balance. I can promote the ideas of the plate in my practice setting.

This is relevant to Practice Effectively as part of the code.

Example 2: Prevention of ill health, reflecting on practice.
I accompanied a patient to a mammography and stayed to observe.

> I had no knowledge of this procedure and was unable to give a satisfactory explanation to the patient and, as a consequence, I was unable to prepare her or answer her questions. I felt I let her down.

> I have learned from what I observed and I will find out more about the discomfort and non-invasive procedure to give a better preparation in future.

This is relevant to Promote Professionalism and Trust as part of the code.

Example 3: Health education, reflecting on a conversation.
I carried out the admission assessment on a patient with her family following a recent diagnosis of early dementia.

> I now realise how little people understand about this condition and how only a limited amount of information is retained after such a consultation. I also felt my knowledge was limited.

> I will obtain information for patients and families and ensure that I am more detailed in my assessment of learning needs.

This is relevant to Prioritise People as part of the code.

Example 4: Health protection reflecting on observation.
I observed a primary care consultation when a patient was adamant he should be given antibiotics for his cold.

(Continued)

(Continued)

Listening to the doctor's response made me realise I could not have given a clear reply as I had not read the evidence, although I understood the issue of antibiotic resistance.

I can speak to patients regarding the awareness of this resistance and ensure my practice area records show that the message is being passed on. I will find out about the 'antibiotic guardian'.

This is relevant to Preserve Safety as part of the code.

These are just some brief outlines of how you might go about structuring your reflective writing for health promotion practice.

Activity 8.1   *Reflection*

- How confident are you that you have the ability to develop health-promoting practice skills?

Look back on previous practice experience and see areas where health-promoting practice could have been a feature of your encounter with patients.

- What, action, if any, have you planned to improve these skills for health promotion practice?
- Could you now explain what health promotion is, having read Chapter 1?
- Do you now understand how it fits into public health (see Chapter 6)?

As this activity is based on your own skills development, there is no outline answer at the end of the chapter.

Case study: Reflecting on practice experience and learning resources

Hannah has enjoyed her practice experience in outpatients. There have been many clinics attended and other disciplines to learn from. She thinks back to the diabetes clinic and the time spent with the specialist nurse, diabetologist, podiatrist, dietician and optometrist – all involved in the care of patients with types 1 and 2 diabetes. Hannah was encouraged by her mentor to look at the various teaching materials available to the patients and how they might facilitate patient learning. Hannah remembers that some patients had apps on their smartphones. One enabled calculation of food portion sizes, allowing measurement of carbohydrates. A further app assisted with insulin dose calculation. In their discussion about learning resources, Hannah's mentor points out that, while some health apps for smartphones may indeed play a useful role in health education and have great potential, UK smartphone ownership is at the lowest among older groups and less wealthy people. These are the very people who make up the bulk of patients attending NHS services. Hannah reflects that she must take time to explore the NHS Choices health app library, as there may be resources there for her to update and follow health themes.

Ways of keeping up to date

It makes sense for nurses to develop an understanding of where and how local practice comes about from strategic guidelines and planning. Sometimes you might find yourself having to explain this concept to patients who may think that what is practised locally has been dreamed up by your colleagues, rather than being aware of the fact that public health is set to a standard nationally.

One way of keeping up to date is to read the newspapers, either hard copy or online in the library (or even on a Kindle). The quality broadsheets give more detailed and evidenced-based, in-depth health reports. You may find that the tabloid newspapers only present the views of the reporters and give no references. The in-depth reports that reflect new research, or government health decisions and position statements, can provide topics for you to follow up in your personal updating and continuing development. Often such newspaper reports will give a source for the information, such as a government department or, if it was research, where the original study took place and who has carried it out. In these cases the department can be checked out for further details, or you can carry out a search for the original journal article in which the research was published. Keeping abreast of newspaper health articles is a simple but effective way of maintaining an update. In addition, the news channel websites have health news sections and you can follow reports. You can be sure that patients will read the papers and follow health reports. Often they will save up this information to ask you what you think about the subject! Being able to hold a meaningful evidence-based conversation with patients about current developments, perhaps even correcting a misconception or misunderstanding, is important in establishing a confident and competent manner in day-to-day professional practice.

Activity 8.2   *Reflection*

Think about a past clinical placement and an occasion when you observed or participated in health promotion practice.

- Can you think about how you judged the interaction? What was good about it? What could be improved?
- When you start your next new practice experience, how do you think you could go about preparing for health-promoting practice?
- How will you update your skills and knowledge for health promotion?

As this activity is based on your own skills development, there is no outline answer at the end of the chapter.

All students find that finance can be an issue. Sharing the expense of subscribing to a relevant professional journal can be a way around this. You may have one or two friends, perhaps more, studying on your course, with whom you could get together. This will lead to you all reading and sharing information and topics for health promotion more immediately. Some students choose to form a study group while at university. This can be a gathering together to discuss coursework, for example, but it could also be to discuss aspects of health-promoting practice and to share your experiences with each other. Benefits of peer-assisted study sessions can be time that enables development of analytical skills, and the ability to question and challenge the status quo. Planning time for reading each week is a good habit to develop as a student and, if it becomes a regular event on your schedule, it is likely that you will continue with this style of update in the future as a qualified nurse. Setting aside time for reading may be more of a problem for some students than others, however, but there are ways around this. First, have a plan, and then it's more likely to happen. Gather your material together for reading in the first instance, and sort it into priority order to read. Perhaps you have a commitment to reading for a particular total time each week, let's say one hour; you may choose more time. Break this total time into smaller portions of time. This way you can build it into your schedule. Use your travelling time, for example – you could read on the bus or train. Use your break time to read on placement – get yourself a cup of tea or coffee and settle down to update for 20–30 minutes. Use your time while waiting for appointments or to collect children from school. At university, use your time wisely to access computer time in the library for reading on one particular day of the week. Think of all the small portions of time that you could have used to read and update your knowledge of health promotion, and then you have found a way to keep your practice updated.

To summarise:

- read the quality broadsheet newspapers for health articles;
- share the expense with friends for a subscription to a relevant professional health journal for sharing reading about health promotion;
- form study groups – share with others on your course about health-promoting practice;
- make a plan for reading – plan for time to read each week; build your schedule, for example train or bus journeys, waiting for appointments, waiting to collect children, or a tea break at work; we suggest a total of 60 minutes each week broken up into two or three manageable portions of time.

The following case study gives an overview of a student's response to preparation for a future practice experience. She will have to make a plan to keep updated and explore further skills in health promotion practice.

Case study: Preparing for a practice experience

Eva has just found out that her practice experience will be on the coronary care unit. She has already had a medical ward placement where patients had a mixture of respiratory and cardiac problems. During a tutorial meeting with her personal development tutor, they discussed what prior knowledge and skills Eva can take with her to the next experience. Her personal development tutor has advised that she update herself and prepare with some background reading. In addition to updating her understanding about the anatomy and physiology of the heart, her tutor suggests that she consults the British Heart Foundation (BHF) website, where she will find out about heart health: www.bhf.org.uk.

Eva revisits her CPR (cardio-pulmonary resuscitation) skills notebook, for the study of emergency life support skills, and reminds herself about the signs and symptoms of myocardial infarction. She is

continued . . .

interested to find out from the BHF website that, in the UK, heart disease kills one in three women as well as one in three men. In fact, she discovers that women are three times more likely to die from heart disease than breast cancer, something she had no awareness of. Eva resolves to update herself as much as possible. She makes a plan to consult the links to 'protecting yourself against heart disease', 'lifestyle advice' and 'risk factors' on the BHF website. She also plans to find out the likely health promotion advice patients will be given in preparation for their discharge from hospital, and what kinds of health promotion support they will need afterwards.

Keeping a record of health promotion practice

A *portfolio* is a means of keeping a record of development to analyse and evaluate learning and practice. You will probably have had to compile a portfolio of your undergraduate learning and developments while you are studying at university, reflecting your progress on your nursing programme. Your portfolio will be kept for a number of reasons:

- to record professional development and experience;
- to record your reflection on practice;
- to record a focus on work practices;
- to assist you with organising your learning by recording your future aims and targets.

The information stored within your portfolio should be more than a 'what I have done' list of activities. The contents of the portfolio must have a focus on what you have learned, how you can apply this to practice in the future or how you have applied this to your practice currently. Sometimes students can get lost in their lengthy writing, describing what has happened. They then forget to write or give a very scanty account of what they have learned as a result of the encounter or practice. The balance must be found in explaining what took place, what has been learned and how this may affect future practice, and which, if any, changes may take place as a result of this event. Becoming a health-promoting nurse, creating a culture of health promotion in your practice, is a worthy entry in your portfolio, so record your reflection on your health-promoting practice.

The next case study considers a student's reflection following a new experience with health-promoting practice at a health education event.

Case study: Health-promoting practice

Justin is studying for a top-up degree in nursing. As part of his programme of study he has been able to access a health promotion module at degree level. He finds it very relevant to his current post, which is in practice at a genito-urinary medicine outpatients department (GUM clinic). Part of the formative

(continued)

continued . . .

assessment strategy for the module involves the students working in a team to conduct a health education event, on university premises, in the student union. The event is a health fair led by students (studying on the module with Justin) for students (other undergraduates). This is peer-led health promotion practice. The subject is sexual health education, raising awareness about chlamydia infection. Justin feels that he is up to date with his knowledge about the problems of chlamydia infection, but he finds himself sharing information with the other students in his team and suggests they visit the National Chlamydia Screening Programme website, part of Public Health England, at chlamydiascreening.nhs.uk/ps, for the latest news and updates.

What Justin lacks experience in is participating in the running of a health fair. It will be his first experience of health promotion practice at such an event; there is a lot to learn! He will have to select and prepare resources for the health fair, set up an information stall, capture the attention of fellow students, engage in health conversation and impart information to students. Hopefully, he can encourage screening for chlamydia and get students to take up testing if appropriate.

All of this health-promoting practice can be recorded in his professional portfolio, as he reflects on his learning experiences and sets out his actions for improving his practice.

Future practice

Once you have become a qualified nurse in your area of practice, you will have continued professional guidance for practice from the NMC *Code* (2015). If you find employment in the NHS, your NHS Trust hospital may be following the competence framework to support personal development within the NHS. This is the Knowledge and Skills Framework (KSF) and it was designed to:

- identify the knowledge and skills that you need to apply in your post;
- help guide your development;
- provide a fair and objective framework on which to base review and development for all staff;
- provide the basis for career progression in the NHS (DH, 2004a).

The KSF was designed to promote quality care and support staff and is linked to their pay and career progression (RCN, 2005). Each NHS job has a KSF outline, which describes the knowledge and skills that people are required to have when they apply for a job. This means thinking about your health-promoting skills and how they match the KSF requirements. An independent review commissioned by the NHS Staff Council discovered that there is a variable take-up of the KSF framework due to its complexity. The framework was simplified to make it easier to use and for staff to identify the skills they require to do their job and to determine development needs (see Useful websites).

Once a year, you and your future line manager will review and appraise your performance. If your Trust Hospital is using the framework you can apply your knowledge and skills against the KSF outline. From this process you can then develop a personal development plan (PDP) and this can be kept in your professional portfolio. Some of these development plans could be about you improving on your health-promoting practice skills. The KSF and the development review process are about **lifelong learning**, something that is discussed in a Department of Health policy, *A High Quality Workforce: NHS Next Stage Review* (DH, 2008a), which puts a strong emphasis on linking clinical practice, academic development and the best use of available evidence for enhancing practice. It further acknowledges the fact that the end of any pre-registration nursing programme is not the end of learning, but is the start of lifelong learning. The KSF may therefore be a critical tool for newly qualified nurses in supporting early career development needs, and portfolios will be an essential way of presenting the evidence of your practice and reflection, providing a focus for discussion at the time of the performance review.

Finally, the NMC (2015) explains the requirement of practice for registered nurses, the professional development, education and training of registrants, and their fitness for practice. The revalidation process was updated in 2015. Overall this process should lead to improvement in practice and therefore has public protection benefits. Trained nurses must give evidence of 450 hours of practice, 35 hours of continuing practice development (CPD) and five pieces of reflective practice evidence with further evidence of reflective discussion with another registered practitioner.

All of these structures and guidelines are there to support you in your future practice as a nurse and this will include your health-promoting practice. Your professional portfolio will be different from that of other students because it is about *you*. It should provide evidence of how you have developed personally and professionally. It should give an account of your achievements and these should include health-promoting practice and any PDPs for your future learning. In the above case studies, both Justin and Eva had to reflect on what they already knew, what they are learning through current health-promoting practice and what they need to learn in the future. Finally, they would be able to make development plans for their health-promoting role as nurses.

Chapter summary

This chapter has considered the guidance from the NMC (2015) for continuing with your personal and professional development and keeping your skills updated. It has also explored and suggested some ways of keeping updated for health-promoting practice. By reflecting on health promotion practice carried out, nurses are enabled to make sense from the experiences they encounter. Finally, it has looked at how you can record this activity in your professional portfolio, by exploring and recording new learning, and what you plan to do with it, and setting out action plans for further development.

Further reading

Howatson-Jones, L (2010) *Reflective Practice in Nursing*. Exeter: Learning Matters.

This is a useful text for student nurses, introducing reflection; it gives practical help on using reflection techniques.

Hutchfield, K (2010) *Information Skills for Nursing Students.* Exeter: Learning Matters.

This is a useful text that introduces nursing students to key skills in IT, enabling continuation of academic study and professional development.

Read, S (2011) *Success with Your Professional Portfolio for Nursing Students.* Exeter: Learning Matters.

This is an easy-to-read text that gives a valuable and informative guide to the development of a portfolio. The text usefully focuses on reflective writing.

Useful websites

www.nhsemployers.org/payandcontracts/agendaforchange/ksf/simplified-ksf/pages/simplifiedksf.aspx

This is the simplified KSF framework, which has made it easier to use.

www.nmc-uk.org

This is the Nursing and Midwifery Council website. Use the search box on the NMC home page to access your topic.

Glossary

advocate someone who pleads on behalf of another person or group; in health promotion this involves representing the combined efforts of individuals and groups to gain political and social support for a specific health programme or goal.

affective concerned with an individual's values, beliefs and emotions.

anti-discriminatory treating each person on their own merit without prejudice as to their colour, gender, disability, ethnicity, sexual orientation and social class.

commission to secure health services that are effective and meet the needs of the people and also to provide the best value for the local people and taxpayers.

community development working in and also with the community, aiming to promote better health for the whole community by building local skills and the capacity for the community to develop and evaluate initiatives that aim to improve its health status.

concordance this means that the patient and the nurse enter into a negotiated agreement regarding care, health outcomes and health behaviour based on cooperation rather than on issues of compliance or non-compliance.

continuing professional development the obligation of professionals to keep themselves up to date and competent in theory and practice. This is often provided as compulsory or voluntary programmes of study by employers, professional bodies and universities.

critical consciousness a widely used concept developed by Brazilian educator Paulo Freire. It means that one develops an objective awareness of social, political and economic oppression and takes action against the process of oppression.

cultural competence the ability to work across multiple cultures and successfully meet the health needs of patients from different cultures.

cultural sensitivity this means that one is aware of existing cultural differences and how these differences may have an effect on an individual's behaviour.

demography the study of the statistics about population characteristics, i.e. age, gender, social class, ethnicity and race.

empowering describes a process that enables an individual to take control of his or her own health.

epidemiology the study of the distribution, determinants and control of disease in populations.

equity fairness – the distribution of resources for health on the basis of need.

external locus of control a belief that a range of events in your life is occurring regardless of your own efforts.

health agenda health issues in the media, public or policy domain ranked according to the amount of time, attention and importance they are given in discussion, debate and action.

health behaviour activities undertaken by an individual, regardless of actual or perceived health status, for the purpose of promoting, protecting or maintaining health, whether or not such behaviour is objectively effective towards that end (WHO, 1998).

health gain a measurable improvement in health status, in individuals or a population, attributable to an earlier health intervention.

health improvement the area of public health related to improving the health of the population by, for example, tackling obesity, sexually transmitted infections, alcohol and substance misuse and smoking. Sometimes used as a title for organisational functions or planning documents instead of health promotion.

health outcomes changes in the health status of individuals or of a population as a result of a health promotion intervention.

holistic an approach that addresses all of the dimensions of health and the whole of someone's life.

inequalities in health the gap between the health of different population groups – people from different social classes or ethnic backgrounds, or the better and worse off in our society.

internal locus of control a belief that the course of your life is largely up to you.

lay a term meaning non-professional. It is generally used for patients or community, so the lay viewpoint is that of the patient rather than that of the nurse or other health professional.

life skills abilities to adopt positive behaviours that enable individuals to deal effectively with the demands and challenges of everyday life.

lifelong learning learning activity undertaken throughout life either formally or informally.

lifestyle the sum total of behaviours that make up the way a person lives, including leisure and work.

lobbying direct attempts to influence legislation through direct interaction with politicians – petitions, contacting Members of Parliament, attending public meetings or demonstrating.

long-term condition a condition that does not have a finite duration and currently cannot be cured but can be managed with medication.

NHS local community health services in Wales, Scotland and Northern Ireland this currently means local NHS organisations responsible for managing health services and health promotion/ improvement in the community. In England their NHS functions have been transferred to GP consortia (Primary Care Trusts have gone) and health promotion/improvement has been transferred to local authorities (since April 2013). In Northern Ireland Health and Personal Social Services are provided as one integrated service in 19 Health and Social Services (HSS) Trusts.

In Wales, there are 22 local health boards that cover the same areas as the 22 local authorities. They broadly fulfil the role of the English PCTs.

In Scotland, the NHS is divided into NHS Boards. The role of these Boards is the protection and improvement of the health of their respective residents through implementation of the Health Improvement Programme. Sixty-three PCTs operate within the geographical boundaries of individual NHS Boards.

non-judgemental avoiding the moral judgement of others and of their behaviour.

partnership local collaboration by statutory, voluntary and private sector organisations, communities and individuals in planning, implementing and evaluating health promotion.

pathophysiology the abnormal physiological changes taking place within our bodies due to a disease or an injury.

patient activation is a process that enables a patient to change his/her health behaviour. It involves patient participation and engagement in decision making and management of his/her long term condition.

peer education community programmes in which members of a community or group of people are recruited, trained and supported to carry out health promotion among their peers.

policy a broad statement of principles of how to proceed in relation to a specific issue, i.e. national policy on immigration or housing.

sector organisations are usually classified into three types: public sector, financed by taxation (NHS and local authorities); private sector (business and commerce); and voluntary sector (charities, not-for-profit and voluntary organisations).

self-efficacy belief in one's capabilities to organise and execute the actions required to manage prospective situations.

self-esteem the extent to which a person regards him- or herself to be of value. It is essential for feeling good about yourself and taking independent action.

self-management an enabling process that expands beyond self-care as it encompasses elements of health promotion, namely education, prevention, protection, attitudes, behaviours and skills. It recognises that people with long-term conditions are in charge of their own lives and health. It also acknowledges that they are the primary decision makers about what actions they can take in relation to the management of their own conditions.

social class a measure of a person's position in society.

social exclusion the inability of certain groups or individuals to participate fully in life due to structural inequalities in access to social, economic, political and cultural resources.

social marketing the application of marketing (selling) techniques to achieve social good. In terms of health behaviour, it means attracting people into changing to healthier choices and behaviours.

socio-economic status a way of classifying social class by income levels, or occupations, which have an effect on lifestyles.

strategy a broad plan of actions that specifies what is to be achieved, how and when. It provides a framework for planning.

sustainable in the context of health services, describes the provision of services that maintain the long-term well-being of the population.

telehealth a new way of healthcare delivery using communication technologies. It enables health professionals to provide clinical services remotely as well as non-clinical healthcare such as, for example, health promotion. This is transmitted using available telecommunication infrastructure such as the internet, email, text messaging or Skype.

victim blaming an approach to health education that emphasises individual action and does not address external forces that influence the individual person. In other words, blaming the victim of an illness for not acting to improve his or her health.

References

Acheson, D (1988) *Public Health in England.* London: HMSO.

Acheson, D (1998) *Independent Inquiry into Inequalities in Health Report.* London: The Stationery Office.

Ajzen, I and Fishbein, M (1980) *Understanding Attitudes & Predicting Social Behaviour.* Englewood Cliffs, NJ: Prentice Hall.

Atkin, WS, Edwards, R, Kralj-Hans, I, Wooldrage, K, Hart, A, Northover, JMA, Parkin, DM, Wardle, J, Duffy, SW and Cuzick, J (2010) Once only flexible sigmoidoscopy screening in prevention of colorectal cancer: a multicentre randomised controlled trial. *The Lancet,* 375(9726): 1624–33.

Babor, TF and Higgins-Biddle, JC (2001) *Brief Intervention for Hazardous and Harmful Drinking: A Manual for Use in Primary Care.* Geneva: World Health Organization.

Bandura, A (1977) Self-efficacy: toward a unifying theory of behaviour change. *Psychological Review,* 84: 191–215.

Becker, MH (ed.) (1974) *The Health Belief Model and Personal Health Behaviour.* Thorofare, NJ: Slack.

Better Days Cancer Care (2012) Patient Navigation Launch. Available online at Betterdays.uk.com (last accessed April 2016).

Bloom, BS (1984) *Taxonomy of Educational Objectives. Handbook 1: Cognitive Domain.* Boston, MA: Addison-Wesley.

Bowen, RL, Duffy, SW, Ryan, DA, Hart, IR and Jones, JL (2008) Early onset of breast cancer in a group of British black women. *British Journal of Cancer,* 98: 227–81.

Bradshaw, JR (1972) The concept of social need. *New Society,* 496: 640–3.

British Heart Foundation (2015) *I've Got My Blood Pressure Under Control.* Birmingham, UK: BHF.

Cabe, J, Kirk, S, Nelson, P, Greenwood, D and Bojke, L (2006) *Can Peer Education Influence People with Diabetes?* Final report to the FSA. Available online at www.foodbase.org.uk/admintools/reportdocuments/01–1-449_91_146_EPP_final_report_04–09–06_as_sent.pdf (accessed 20 October 2010).

Cancer Research UK (2008) *Increasing Uptake of NHS Cancer Screening Services: A Screening Matters Report.* London: Cancer Research UK.

Cancer Research UK (2010) Science Update Blog. Available online at http://scienceblog.cancerresearchuk.org/2010/04/28/new-study-marks-major-advance-in-bowel-cancer (accessed 4 July 2010).

Cancer Research UK (2014a) *Breast Cancer in Men.* London: Cancer Research UK.

Cancer Research UK (2014b) *Screening for Prostate Cancer.* London: Cancer Research UK.

Cancer Research UK (2014c) *A Study Looking at Screening for Men Who are at an Increased Risk of Developing Prostate Cancer* (IMPACT). London: Cancer Research.

Cummings, J (2016) *Leading Change, Adding Value: A Framework for Nursing, Midwifery and Care Staff.* NHS England 05247. Available online at: https://www.england.nhs.uk/wp-content/uploads/2016/05/nursing-framework.pdf (accessed 10 October 2016).

Day, M (2013) *Breast Cancer Risk for British Asian Women.* Presentation at the Cancer Outcomes Conference, National Cancer Centre Intelligence Network, Brighton, 12–14 June.

Department of Health (DH) (1992) *The Health of the Nation: A Strategy for Health in England.* London: HMSO.

Department of Health (DH) (1999) *Saving Lives: Our Healthier Nation.* London: HMSO.

Department of Health (DH) (2001) *National Service Framework for Diabetes: Standards*. London: Department of Health.

Department of Health (DH) (2003) *Toolkit for Producing Patient Information*. London: Department of Health. Available online at http://www.dh.gov.uk/en/Publicationsandstatistics/Publications/PublicationsPolicy AndGuidance/DH_4070141 (accessed 19 June 2010).

Department of Health (DH) (2004a) *The NHS Knowledge and Skills Framework and the Development Review Process*. London: Department of Health.

Department of Health (DH) (2004b) *Choosing Health: Making Healthier Choices Easier Choices*. London: Department of Health.

Department of Health (DH) (2006) *Our Health, Our Care, Our Say*. London: Department of Health.

Department of Health (DH) (2007) *Health Literacy*. London: Department of Health.

Department of Health (DH) (2008a) *A High Quality Workforce: NHS Next Stage Review*. London: Department of Health.

Department of Health (DH) (2008b) *High Quality Care for All: The Next Stage Review Final Report*. London: Department of Health.

Department of Health (DH) (2009) *Your Health Your Way: A Guide to Long-term Conditions and Self-care*. London: Department of Health.

Department of Health (DH) (2010a) *Improving the Health and Wellbeing of People with Long-term Conditions*. London: Department of Health.

Department of Health (DH) (2010b) *Healthy Lives, Healthy People: Our Strategy for Public Health in England*. London: Department of Health.

Department of Health (DH) (2011) *National Quality Board Advice and Recommendations*. London: Department of Health.

Department of Health (DH) (2012a) *Health and Social Care 2012*. London: Department of Health. Available online at www.legislation.gov.uk/ukpga_20120007_en.pdf (accessed 15 July 2016).

Department of Health (DH) (2012b) *NHS Mandate*. London: Department of Health. Available online at www.gov.uk/goverment/publications/the-nhs-mandate (accessed 4 May 2013).

Department of Health (DH) (2013) *A Framework for Sexual Health Improvement in England*. London: Department of Health.

Department of Health and Social Security (DHSS) (1980) *Inequalities in Health: Report of a Research Working Group*. London: DHSS.

Duffy, S, Tabar, L, Olsen, A, Vitak, B, Allgood, P, Chen, T, Yen, A and Smith, R (2010) Absolute numbers of lives saved and overdiagnosis in breast cancer screening, from a randomized trial and from the Breast Screening Programme in England. *Journal of Medical Screening*, 17(1): 25–30.

European Cancer Organisation (ECCO) (2016) Major differences between male and female breast cancer uncovered, but male patients still disadvantaged by lack of research, 10th European Breast Cancer Conference, March. Brussels: ECCO. Available online at https://www.ecco-org.eu/Global/News/ EBCC/EBCC10-PR/2016/03/Major-differences-between-male-and-female-breast-cancers-uncovered (last accessed April 2016).

Gok, M, Heidman, D, van Kemenade, FJ, Berkhof, J, Rozendaal, L, Spruyt, J, Voorhurst, F, Belein, J, Babovic, M, Snijers, P and Meijer, C (2010) HPV testing on self-collected cervicovaginal lavage specimens as screening method for women who do not attend cervical screening: cohort study. *British Medical Journal*, 340: c1040. Available online at www.bmj.com/content/340/bmj.c1040 (accessed 6 June 2013).

Hardyman, R, Hardy, P, Brodie, J and Stephens, R (2005) It's good to talk: comparison of a telephone helpline and website for cancer information. *Patient Education and Counseling*, 57(3): 315–20.

HM Government (2016a) *The National Living Wage: A Step Up for Britain* - HM Government UK. Available on: https://www.livingwage.gov.uk (accessed 15 July 2016).

HM Government (2016b) *Childhood Obesity: A Plan for Action*. Available online at: www.gov.uk/government/uploads/system/uploads/attachment_data/file/546588/ (accessed 8 September 2016).

Hibbart, JH and Cunnningham, PJ (2008) How engaged are consumers in their health and health care, and why does it matter? *Health System Change Research Briefs*, no8, pp1–9. Available online at: www.hschange.com/CONTENT/1019 (accessed on 22 July 2016).

Hibbart, J and Gilburt, H (2014) *Supporting People to Manage their Health. An Introduction to Patient Activation*. London: The King's Fund.

Iddo, G and Prigat, A (2004) Why organisations continue to create patient information leaflets with readability and usability problems: an exploratory study. *Health Education Research*, 20(4): 485–93.

Jacobs, I, Menton, U, Ryan, A et al. (2015) Ovarian cancer screening and mortality in the UK collaborative trial of ovarian cancer screening (UKCTOCS): a randomised control trial. *The Lancet*, March, vol. 387, no.10022: 945 – 956.

Kopans, D (2010) Screening for breast cancer among women in their 40s. *The Lancet Oncology*, 11(12): 1108–9.

Landy, R, Birke, H, Castanon, A and Sasieni, P (2014) Benefits and harm of cervical screening from age 20 years compared with screening from age 25 years. *British Journal of Cancer*, April 12, 110 (7) 1841–6 doi:10. 1038/bjc2014.65

Lorig, K, Mazonson, P and Holman, HR (1993) Evidence suggesting that health education for self-management in patients with chronic arthritis has sustained health benefits while reducing health care costs. *Arthritis and Rheumatism*, 36(4): 439–46.

Marmot, M (2010) *Fair Society, Healthy Lives: Strategic Review of Health Inequalities in England* (The Marmot Review). Available online at www.marmotreview.org (accessed 9 January 2011).

Marmot, M, Altman, D, Cameron, D, Dewar, J, Thompson, S and Wilcox, M (2013) The benefits and harms of breast cancer screening, an independent review. *British Journal of Cancer*, 108(11): 2205–40.

Mencap Accessibility Team (2008) *Make it Clear: A Guide to Easy Read Information*. London: Mencap.

Mukhtar, T, Yeates, D and Goldacre, M (2013) Breast cancer mortality trends in England and the assessment of the effectiveness of mammography screening: population-based study. *Journal of the Royal Society of Medicine*, 106(6): 234–42.

National Health Service (NHS) (2010) *Patient Information*. London: NHS. Available online at www.nhs.uk/tools-and-resources/patient-information (accessed 9 November 2010).

National Health Service (NHS) (2014) *Choices: Abdominal Aortic Aneurysm Screening*. Available online at http://www.nhs.uk/Conditions/abdominal-aortic-aneurysm-screening/Pages/Introduction.aspx (accessed April 2016).

National Health Service (NHS) (2016) *Screening Programme, Abdominal Aortic Aneurysm Programme, Nurse Specialist Best Practice Guidelines*. London: PHE Publications, NHS.

National Health Service (NHS) Choices (2016) *'Exercise-labels' Should be Added to Food Packets, Expert Argues – Health News*. London: NHS England. Available online at http://www.nhs.uk/news/2016/04April/Pages/Exercise-labels-should-be-added-to-food-packets-expert-argues.aspx (accessed 17 July 2016).

National Health Service England (2014) *Five Year Forward View*. London: NHS England. Available online at https://www.england.nhs.uk (accessed on 25 July 2016).

National Health Service England (2016) *Enhancing the Quality of Life for People Living with Long-term Conditions.* London: NHS England. Available online at https://www.england.nhs.uk/resources/resources-for-ccgs/out-fwrk/dom-2 (accessed on 25 July 2016).

National Institute for Health and Care Excellence (NICE) (2007) *Behaviour Change at Population, Community and Individual Levels.* Public Health Guidance 6. London: NICE.

National Primary Care Research and Development Centre (2007) *National Evaluation of the Expert Patients Programme. Key Findings (Research into Expert Patients – Outcomes in a Randomised Trial)*, Executive Summary 44, March. Manchester, UK: National Primary Care Research and Development Centre. Available online at www.npcrdc.ac.uk/r5.25 (accessed on 17 July 2016).

Naylor, C, Parsonage, M, McDaid, D, Knapp, M, Fossey, M and Galea, A (2012) *Long-term Conditions and Mental Health: The Cost of Co-morbidities.* London: The King's Fund and Centre for Mental Health.

Nightingale, F (1859) *Notes on Nursing: What It Is and What It Is Not* (2007 edition). Radford, VA: Wilder Publications.

Nursing and Midwifery Council (NMC) (2010) *Standards for Pre-registration Nursing Education.* London: NMC.

Nursing and Midwifery Council (NMC) (2015) *The Code: Professional Standards of Practice and Behavior for Nurses and Midwives.* London: NMC.

Office for National Statistics (2015) *Internet Access: Households and Individuals.* Available online at www.onsgov.uk/ons/rel/rdit2/Internet-access-households-and-individuals/2015/index.html (accessed June 2015).

Office of the Public Guardian (2009) *Making Decisions: A Guide for Family, Friends and Other Unpaid Carers: The Mental Capacity Act* (4th edn). London: OPG.

Prime Minister's Commission on the Future of Nursing and Midwifery in England (2010) *Front Line Care.* London: COI.

Prochaska, JO and DiClemente, CC (1982) Transtheoretical therapy: toward a more integrative model of change. *Psychotherapy: Theory Research and Practice,* 20: 161–73.

Public Health Wales (2013) *Report into Measles Outbreak,* published 12 November. Available online at www.wales.nhs.uk/sitesplus/888/news/29688 (accessed 4 December 2013).

Richmond Group of Charities (2016) *Live Longer, Live Well. How We can Achieve the World Health Organization's '25 by 25' Goals in the UK. A Report by the Richmond Group of Charities.* London: Richmond Group of Charities, June. Available online at www.richmondgroupofcharities.org.uk/publications (accessed 5 September 2016).

Rollnick, S, Miller, WR and Butler, CC (2008) *Motivational Interviewing in Health Care: Helping Patients Change Behaviour.* New York: Guilford Press.

Rotter, JB (1966) Generalised expectancies for internal and external control of reinforcement. *Psychological Monographs,* 80(609): 1–28.

Royal College of Nursing (RCN) (2005) *NHS Knowledge and Skills Framework: Outlines for Nursing Posts. RCN Guidance for Nurses and Managers in Creating KSF Outlines in the NHS.* London: RCN.

Royal College of Nursing (RCN) (2012) *Going Upstream: Nursing's Contribution to Public Health.* London: RCN.

Royal National Institute of Blind People (RNIB) (2004) *See It Right Pack.* London: RNIB.

Salem, DS, Kamal, RM, Mandour, SM, Salah, LA and Wessam, R (2013) Breast imaging in the young: the role of MRI in breast cancer screening, diagnosis and follow up. *Journal of Thoracic Disease,* June (suppl.1) S9 – S18, doi;10.3978/j.issn.2072-1439.2013.0502.

Screening.nhs.uk (accessed June 2016).

Self Care Forum (2013) *Save our NHS: Time for Action on Self Care.* London: Self Care Forum.Available online at www.selfcareforum.org/ 2013/10/09/mandate-for-self-care (accessed 4 December 2013).

Tannahill, A (1985) What is health promotion? *Health Education Journal*, 44: 167–8.

Tannahill, A (2009) Health promotion: the Tannahill model revisited. *Public Health*, 123: 396–9.

Tones, BK and Tilford, S (2001) *Health Promotion: Effectiveness, Efficiency and Equity* (3rd edn). Cheltenham: Stanley Thornes.

UK National Screening Committee (UK NSC) (2014) *The Handbook for Vascular Risk Assessment, Risk Reduction and Risk Management* (Updated). Leicester, UK: University of Leicester and UK Screening Committee.

UK National Screening Committee (UK NSC) (2015) UK screening portal. Available online at: https://www.gov.uk/government/publications/uk-national-screening-committee-recommendations-annual-report (accessed 5 July 2016).

Waller, J, Jackowska, M, Marlow, L and Wardle, J (2012) Exploring age differences in reasons for non attendance for cervical screening in a qualitative study. *British Journal of Obstetrics and Gynecology*, 119, 26–32, doi:10.1111/j.1471-0528.2011.03030.x.epubjun14

Wanless, D (2002) *Securing Our Future Health: Taking a Long-term View – An Independent Review*. London: HM Treasury.

Weller, DP and Campbell, C (2009) Uptake in cancer screening programmes: a priority in cancer control. *British Journal of Cancer*, 101(S2): S55–9.

Whitehead, M (1988) *The Health Divide*. London: Penguin.

Williams, B, Poulter, NR, Brown, MJ, Davis, M, McInnes, GT, Potter, JF, Sever, PS and Thom, S McG (2004) Guidelines for management of hypertension: report of the fourth working party of the British Hypertension Society, 2004–BHS IV. *Journal of Human Hypertension*, 18(3): 139–85.

World Health Assembly (1998) *Health-for-all Policy for the Twenty-first Century* (Resolution WHA51.7). Geneva: World Health Organization. Available online at http://dataplan.info/cb21/archiv/material/world healthdeclaration.pdf (accessed 7 May 2010).

World Health Organization (WHO) (1948) *Constitution of the World Health Organization*. Geneva: WHO. Available online at www.who.int/governance/eb/who_constitution_en.pdf (accessed 7 July 2010).

World Health Organization (WHO) (1978) *Primary Health Care: The Alma Ata Conference*. Geneva: WHO. Available online at www.who.int/hpr/NPH/docs/declaration_almaata.pdf (accessed 7 July 2010).

World Health Organization (WHO) (1981) *Global Strategy for Health for All by the Year 2000*. Geneva: WHO. Available online at whqlibdoc.who.int/publications/9241800038.pdf (accessed 8 July 2010).

World Health Organization (WHO) (1986) *The Ottawa Charter*, First International Conference on Health Promotion, 21 November. Geneva: WHO. Available online at: http://www.who.int/healthpromotion/conferences/previous/ottawa/en (accessed 3 May 2013).

World Health Organization (WHO) (1988) *Adelaide Recommendations on Healthy Public Policy*. Geneva: WHO. Available online at: http://www.who.int/healthpromotion/conferences/previous/adelaide/en/index.html (accessed 4 May 2013).

World Health Organization (WHO) (1991) *Sundsvall Statement on Supportive Environments for Health*, Third International Conference on Health Promotion, Sundsvall, 9–15 June. Geneva: WHO. Available online at: www.who.int/healthpromotion/conferences/previous/sundsvall/en (accessed 5 May 2013).

World Health Organization (WHO) (1997) *Jakarta Declaration on Leading Health Promotion into the 21st Century*, Fourth International Conference on Health Promotion, Jakarta, 21–25 July. Geneva: WHO. Available online at: www.who.int/healthpromotion/conferences/previous/jakarta/declaration/en (accessed 6 May 2013).